Praise for *The 100 Plus Club: Livi*

MW01236224

"I found the articles by Paul Dudley White, MD t͟ quotes from Dr. White are very insightful: 'Walk more, eat less, sleep more' and 'A vigorous five mile walk will do more good for an unhappy but otherwise healthy adult than all the medicine and psychology in the world.' I feel that Dr. White was spot on. 21st century cardiology practice could have very well led Uncle Charlie to an earlier death."
-ROBERT GOLDMAN, MD, ATLANTA, GA

"The vast bulk of the book is very detailed, very interesting and beautifully written chapters on Uncle Charlie…readers will be drawn to his compelling story and what could be learned from it more than the typical how-to book with some anecdotal examples. Most people should end up highly motivated after finishing the book and will naturally wonder, 'Now what do I DO' or 'How do I get involved?'"
-BRIAN DYER, USAF Lt/COL (RET'D) NASA, HOUSTON, TEXAS

"This is a true story for the ages of amazing achievement…by living day to day, choice by choice, long and well. I found the author's story in *The 100 Plus Club* as interesting and important as Great Uncle Charlie's. The facts are well stated, quite comprehensive and interesting, making the reader very eager to continue on to learn more."
-NANCY SEPHTON, BERKELEY, CALIFORNIA

"*The 100 Plus Club* is a warm and wonderful read. Fifty-six years after his passing, we are still reading and talking about Great Uncle Charlie. We would all be fortunate to have such a legacy. The front cover is spot on when it says *Living Long and Living Well*. I think Josh Batchelder may have more in common with Great Uncle Charlie than he realizes."
-BRUCE FITZGERALD, COLLEGE PROFESSOR, WASHINGTON, GEORGIA

"This guide is a gateway to experiences and abundance of quality living for yourself and family, while you add years to enjoy it all."
-STEPHEN BARGERON, CFP, KENNESAW, GEORGIA

"This fascinating book is full of a centenarian's wisdom for all ages—about how to design and carry out a successful family and business life that will be to the benefit of my children and grandchildren.'
-GREGG O'NEIL, BUSINESS OWNER, DUNWOODY, GEORGIA

Also by Josh Batchelder

The Wheel: The Art of Wheel and Handwriting Analyses and Quick & Insightful Personality Profiling, Co-authored with Ernest F. Pecci, MD

Personality Profiling in 90 Seconds

Handwriting Reveals You

Military Memoirs about Flying:

Black Watch Diary — A Sequel

Black Watch Diary

Climb to 8 and Wait — If You Can Get Her in the Air, She'll Get You There

the
100 PLUS
CLUB

Living Long and Living Well

Copyright © 2014 - Josh Batchelder

ALL RIGHTS RESERVED - No part of this book may be reproduced in any form or by any electronic or mechanical means, including information storage and retrieval systems, without permission in writing from the authors, except by a reviewer who may quote brief passages in a review.

Cover photo by Dennis Jarvis
Cover design and text layout by Mark Babcock

Published by Deeds Publishing
Marietta, GA
www.deedspublishing.com

Printed in The United States of America

Library of Congress Cataloging-in-Publications Data is available upon request.

ISBN 978-1-941165-17-1

Books are available in quantity for promotional or premium use. For information, write
Deeds Publishing, PO Box 682212, Marietta, GA 30068 or
info@deedspublishing.com.

Josh Batchelder
Military Memoirs
Graphologist Services
PO Box 450525
Atlanta GA 31145

joshgraphologist@bellsouth.net
(770) 621-9000

www.quickprofiling.com
www.blackwatchdiary.com

Second Edition, 2014

10 9 8 7 6 5 4 3 2 1

Josh Batchelder

the
100 PLUS
CLUB
Living Long and Living Well

JOSH BATCHELDER with SALLY A. WALKER

Lakeside, Class 2024
congratulations. Tim,
Now live long + live well
and prosper with your
spiritual life.

Josh

Contents

Acknowledgements

GEORGE SCOTT, ATLANTA WRITERS Club member who coordinates book signings and talks. George, who works for Books for Less, has been tremendously helpful with his guidance, which included slowing down the process to produce a creditable product. George knows how to produce a book that is saleable and the public will appreciate.

Sally A. Walker checked my facts every step of the way, being more objective and making numerous suggestions about choice of words, paragraph positions, etc. She added a younger person's and woman's perspective, and took pictures like a true photo-journalist.

Cousin Doris Tufts Heinold of Wellesley, Massachusetts, presented us with her deceased mother's scrapbook with a wealth of information for the celebrated centenarian period of Uncle Charlie's life (1950-1958). It contains articles and pictures from the Boston Globe and Boston Herald Newspapers, other local and national publications, congratulatory telegrams, and church documents including the program for Uncle Charlie's 100 year commemorative service.

Nancy Elizabeth Batchelder Sephton, of Berkeley, California, is my very special sister, fellow author and supporter. She's taken many hours to fill in her account of accompanying Uncle Charlie to the September, 1953 Republican Club Dinner for President Eisenhower. Nancy provided pictures and memories of Uncle Charlie, and coordinated my visit to Berkeley to consult with medium Tom Flynn.

Donald Richard Batchelder, my twin brother, provided his account of time spent with Uncle Charlie and his perspective regarding Elizabeth "Lizzie" Harris Houghton's tragic death and how that impacted him.

Lisa H. Fagerstrom is the church historian for Harvard-Epworth United Methodist Church. In spite of having a busy schedule, she took time to give us a church tour and give us an account of how Uncle Charlie's service and financial support has impacted the church's history to this day.

Tom Flynn, medium from the UK, contacted Uncle Charlie's spirit which provided encouragement and his current opinions featured in Chapter X "Finishing Touches" 16 May 2013. Uncle Charlie communicated through Tom that he wants his life to be remembered.

Charles Wesley Thiery. Whether proper or not, I thank him for being my mentor and inspiration to live long and live well. I'm amazed at the depth of my lifelong interest and memory of the lessons he taught me. I have been re-energized during the past two and one-half years, improving my eating and exercise habits, to reset my life expectancy target to 105 years.

Tom Millin, retired IBM executive. My tech guru is more than a neighbor; he's also the webmaster for the Atlanta Braves 400 Fan Club. Tom has come quickly to resolve my computer problems, a critically important skill to keep things on track to get this book out! It's hard to over-appreciate his contribution.

Kara M. Jackman, Archivist and Research Collections Librarian of the Boston University School of Theology Library.

Kathleen L. "Kit" Rawlins of the Cambridge Historical Commission.

Louise Ambler, Historian of Christ Church Cambridge—Harvard Square.

James Capobianco, Reference Librarian, Harvard College Library, Harvard University.

Andrea Cronin of The Massachusetts Historical Society.

The Cambridge Historical Society

The Cambridge Public Library

Last but not least, my wife, Betty Ann Sage, the wise one. She's put up with interruptions in family life and trips to Boston, Massachusetts and San Francisco, California to obtain material for this book to bring Uncle Charlie back to life.

Dedication

To my aunt, the late Florence "Marie" Batchelder Tufts for assembling a scrapbook filled with news stories, pictures, telegrams and other documents about Charles Wesley Thiery, AKA Uncle Charlie, 1850-1958.

And to my cousin, Doris Tufts Heinold, for gifting the above scrapbook that enriched our efforts to shine a search light some six decades back to the 1950s; then, that information took us back to the early 1800s.

Finally, to my beautiful and loving sister, Nancy Elizabeth Batchelder Sephton. She contributed many pictures, memories and observations of our family connections to Uncle Charlie.

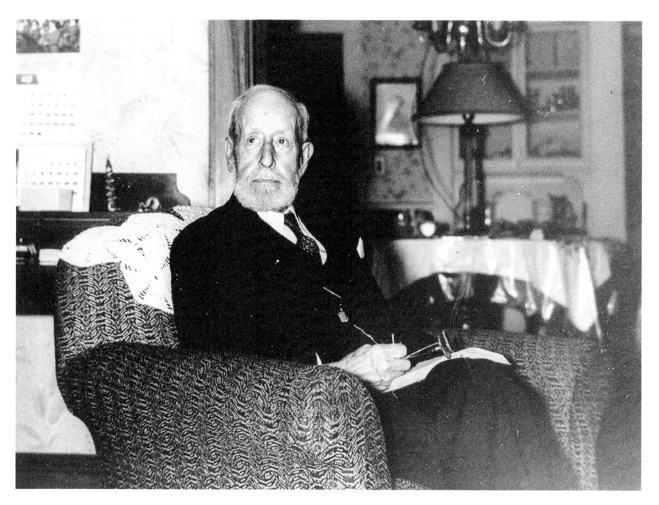

Foreword: Josh

EXTENDING LONGEVITY SEEMS TO be all the rage today. Charles Wesley Thiery (1850-1958), AKA my Great Uncle Charlie (UC), is my inspiration for *living long and living well*. My lifelong journey to age one hundred plus began when I first met him.

He was about 89 years old and I was eight when I recall being fascinated by his presence and stories. Uncle Charlie had a trim white beard, and often a skull-cap on his bald head. Usually, I saw him wearing a white shirt and tie, and a gold chain leading to his tailored suit's vest pocket watch. He was a wiry 5 feet 3 inches in stature and his voice was gruff. Frequently he'd reach for his white handkerchief or Kleenex

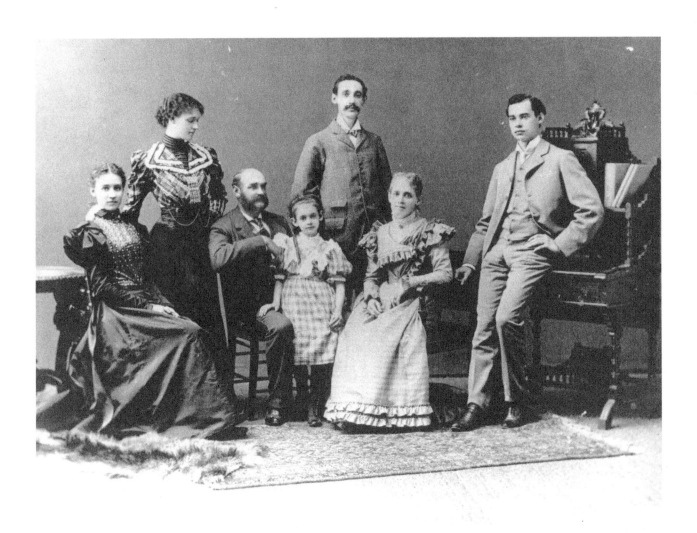

The Batchelder Family circa 1900

to wipe his nose. It was said, to save money, he'd tear a tissue into four pieces. Uncle Charlie's shiny black leather low quarter shoes had triangular holes cut above his toes. At age 82, I know. I wear New Balance shoes that breathe and prevent pain from heat swelling my toe joints. He told me, "I walk a vigorous mile a day and have warm milk and crackers before I retire. Eat breakfast like a king, lunch like a prince, and dinner like a pauper."

One of his stories I remember well was about a business situation with a lesson to be learned from the proper pricing of goods for sale. He acquired a large quantity of very low cost diamonds from overseas. He proceeded to mount the diamonds, as a jobber, and distributed the rings to retail stores. At low prices, the shops expected to sell them quickly. However, they didn't move. He suggested his retailers raise their prices to approximate the price of similar diamond rings. Rapidly, they sold out. Obviously, buyers were suspicious of the value at the lower price.

My father, John Thiery Batchelder, a Harvard educated attorney, was Uncle Charlie's nephew. They attended weekly Boston Republican Party luncheons. They often went to movies. They shared a mutual love of reading. Uncle Charlie was a Sunday school teacher for three decades. Did that encourage Father to read the entire Bible three times? August 1947, my father passed. He was a month shy of his 70th birthday and Uncle Charlie was in his 97th year. Consequently, my challenge, as an adult, became extrapolating back to better understand the work and personal worlds of Uncle Charlie and my father.

For the next few years, my widowed mother, Emma Macaulay Batchelder, a nurse, had regular contact with Uncle Charlie. She was the beneficiary of my father's share of

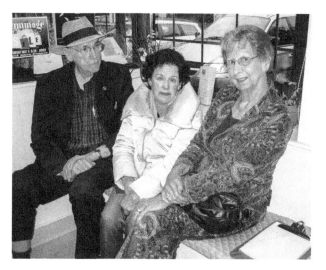

Josh, left, Doris, center, Betty Ann, right

Uncle Charlie's estate. During 1950, in a staircase fall, my mother, nearing age 60, suffered a broken leg. Confined to a wheelchair, she still had to manage two live-in elderly patients. She seized an opening to occupy a two floor apartment next to Uncle Charlie's. Sister Nancy temporarily left college to serve as caretaker for Mother and her patients. Sister Joan and twin brother, Donald, also occupied this same apartment for six months while they were attending Boston University. In the last few years of Uncle Charlie's life, they got to know him better. During this same period, I was married with three children and a full time Harvard University student on the GI

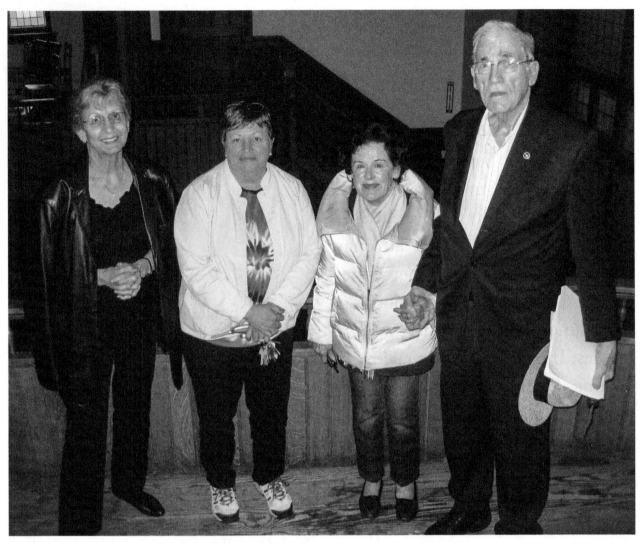

Betty Ann, Lisa Fagerstrom, Doris, Josh

Bill. I also flew part time with the Air National Guard out of Logan Airport Boston and Grenier Air Force Base, Manchester, New Hampshire. As a result, I missed regular contact with Uncle Charlie. My siblings, Nancy and Donald, gave me their accounts of his final years. They accompanied Uncle Charlie to church services and dined with him. They became prime sources for my adult understanding of this extraordinary human being—an active, successful, and dedicated Christian gentleman.

May of 2012 my cousin, Doris Tufts Heinold, Uncle Charlie's grandniece, gifted me with her mother Marie's (Uncle Charlie's niece and my father's sister) scrapbook. It is filled with seven and one half years' worth of newspaper stories and pictures about Uncle Charlie from Boston and across the United States, Germany, and Japan. It is a goldmine. It recounts the celebrated centenarian's early life, businesses, church, and civic activity. It has reflections of his Civil War service. He enlisted in the 1st Brigade Cavalry of the Boston Light Dragoons. In an October, 1950 feature story by Alta Maloney, "The centenarian has another proud memory; that of being a corporal at age 17 in the state Cavalry." Handwriting analysis has enabled me to validate family and news stories of Uncle Charlie's values, opinions, and behavior; in short, a number of realistic portraits. All of this exploration resulted in more questions.

Uncle Charlie's early inspiration enabled me to travel a parallel path of growing old and living well; this has helped me understand and appreciate him more than ever.

Chapter X (Finishing Touches) was an effort to find more evidence of his military and personal life. The FBI and police have used

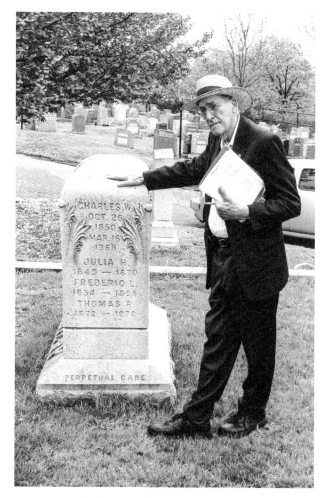

*Josh at the Thiery family plot
Cambridge Cemetery, May 2012*

mediums to find missing evidence that cracked cases thought to be unsolvable. In fact, in Uncle's Charlie's family, a medium indicated where the gun was located (under a stairway) that "fingered" the murderer.

We travelled to Cambridge, Massachusetts May, 2012, to meet with Ms. Lisa Fagerstrom, the Harvard Epworth Methodist Church historian.

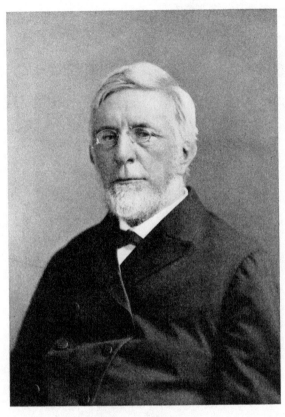

HENRY O. HOUGHTON
From a Painting in Cambridge City Hall

Portrait of Henry Houghton,
Carmichael Art Conservation photo,
Cambridge Historical Commission

Pictures were taken of Uncle Charlie's birth home in Cambridge and last home in Belmont, Massachusetts. We visited and took pictures of the Thiery family gravesite plot at the Cambridge Municipal Cemetery.

Mid July, 2013, I returned to the Boston area to Cousin Doris' home to see if the medium, Tom Flynn's, hints of the location of missing doc-

uments would prove helpful. I went to the Boston University archives looking for United Methodist Church connections of Uncle Charlie and the Henry Oscar Houghton family. Henry Oscar was the founder of Houghton-Mifflin publishing company. Finally, I visited the Harvard University Houghton Library to discover possible links between Uncle Charlie and the Houghton family.

Co-author, "Savvy" Sally A. Walker, and my wife, Betty Ann Sage, "The-Wise-One" motored with me to Scituate, south shore from Boston, to seek a Master Graphoanalyst's personality profile of Uncle Charlie. Eileen Page, MGA, completed a comprehensive evaluation of Uncle Charlie which appears in Chapter XI. He is the textbook perfectionist. Eileen is the author of the book *The Paradox of Perfection.* Since my wife and Sally are two more perfectionists, it proved to be a very insightful exchange.

Back in Atlanta, a google search turned up President Eisenhower's cardiologist, Paul Dudley White,

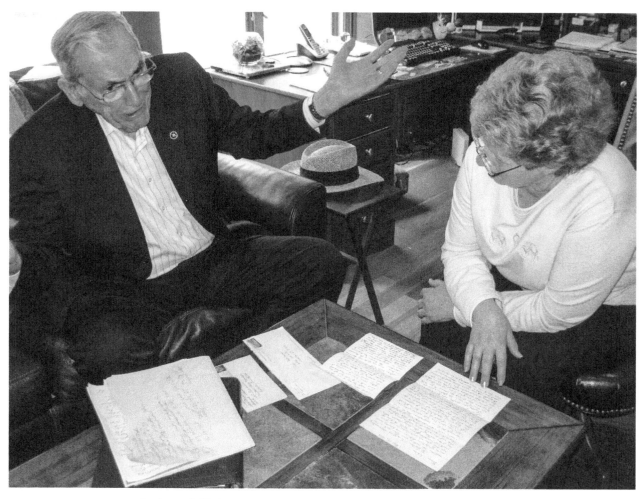

Josh with Eileen Page examining Uncle Charlie's 1956 letters

MD's, detailed account of his medical observations of Uncle Charlie from 1950—1958—his exemplar for medical societies on how to extend longevity. Dr. White's report (Chapter III) validates what our family witnessed, heard about and believed concerning Uncle Charlie's lifestyle and health.

A copy of his 1952 Last Will and Testament (Chapter V) tells the story of his values and his care for relatives and good causes, including the Harvard-Epworth United Methodist Church. He distributed his wealth to a long list of worthy, charitable bequests before the remainder was left to nieces and nephews and their survivors. It is a telling testimonial of a legend to be remembered. Our key technique to explore Uncle Charlie's personality

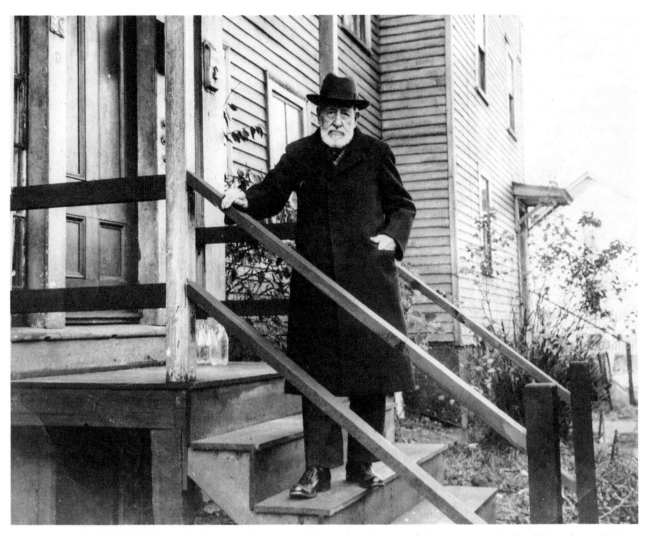

Uncle Charlie's original (birth) home on Tremont Street in Cambridge, Massachusetts

has been using handwriting analysis. It enabled us to validate or question all the available information about Uncle Charlie. We found him to be honest. His signatures tell us that he was true to what he represented himself to be. We obtained added understanding of the intense emotional pressures Uncle Charlie had to deal with. What about his con-

version to Christianity at age 15? It provided structure to help him cope with life.

Analysis of my handwriting shows that I share much of his basic emotional depth and empathy for others. However, I've experienced living in many more environments than Uncle Charlie did. I mean adapting to many states, climates, and organizations. In spite of these differences, I've sought to emulate many of his strategies to succeeding over a long lifetime.

Many questions remain to be answered in spite of what we now know from all of our sources regarding Uncle Charlie. Why did he remain a lifelong bachelor? How close was he, really, to Henry Oscar Houghton's daughter, Elizabeth, "Lizzie" Harris Houghton? How involved were they at church, work, and philanthropy? What are the details about his reported eight years of service in the Massachusetts State Militia Cavalry, the 1st Brigade, Boston Light Dragoons? About 1941, why did he move from his original Tremont Street, Cambridge residence to 121 Hammond Road, Belmont?

Like a detective trying to find missing pieces of evidence, I went to Berkeley, California, to consult a heralded English Medium, Tom Flynn. During our lengthy session Tom captured Uncle Charlie's words and feelings. They validated our known facts and suggested places to search

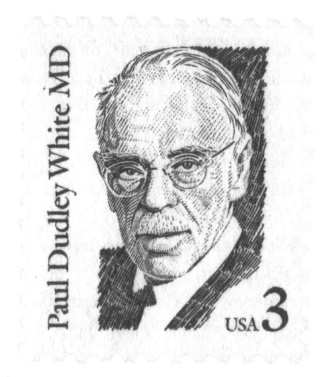

The United States Post Office issued a 100th birthday anniversary stamp in 1986 for Dr. White.

for more answers in Wellesley, Belmont, and Cambridge.

In Chapter II, I list 47 dominate character traits of Uncle Charlie. In a two page letter he wrote at age 106, each writing stroke source of these traits is identified. He was a diligent worker, perfectionist/procrastinator always striving to succeed.

Chapter III, Paul Dudley White, MD, the late, prominent Boston cardiologist, provided his post demise medical findings and lifestyle report about Uncle Charlie. He served as President Dwight David Eisenhower's personal physician. He described Uncle Charlie as having "the heart of a boy." But you need to remember Uncle Charlie's wisdom, "the strong die before the weak." Derive your own theories as you follow him dealing with his new celebrity status. Imagine how you would feel after four years of being a country wide celebrated centenarian. I believe his becoming a star contributed to Uncle Charlie's uncharacteristic and unconventional marriage proposal at age 104 to my sister, Nancy, his grandniece.

You'll read about Uncle Charlie's daily routine and public life. As you learn about his lifestyle and behavior, you'll compare his healthy habits extending longevity with pockets of cultures around-the-world that have more centenarians and super centenarians (110 plus). The book, *The Blue Zones* by Dan Buettner, describes nine lessons for living longer from the people who've lived the longest. For years, I've sought out the latest and best findings regarding living long and living well. Un-

cle Charlie exemplified seven of our eight healthy habits. The eighth, for him, a teetotaler, was not an option:

1. Exercise daily, be active! Walk up the stairs instead of taking the elevator, park further away from shops and stores.

2. Diet, what we ingest. Plenty of salad greens and fresh vegetables. No drug abuse or cigarettes. Light meals, especially at night.

3. Stress reduction. Daily quiet time, plenty of sleep, and laugh a lot. Live in the moment as much as possible. Soldiers on the battle field facing death 24/7 don't contemplate their possible demise. They live in-the-moment, and strive to complete the mission. One of my hatha yoga instructors, Mr. Tim Geoghegan, said, "Meditation is not doing anything. It's a preparation to do something. If all we do is meditate, we don't need to be on the face of the earth."

4. Connections. Maintain closeness to family, friends, and companions—pets, too!

5. A spiritual/purposeful life. Discover why you're on the face of the earth. What lessons are you learning?

6. Grow your brain. Stimulate yours by learning something new, take on a new hobby, study a different language, etc. We now know you can learn at all ages.

7. Read, read, read. You'll learn to solve more problems and stay more positive than watching the daily madness on TV.

8. Imbibe a small glass or two a day of quality red wine. Uncle Charlie was a teetotaler.

While the principal purpose of the *100 Plus Club* book is to illustrate habits of those living long and living well, there are a few intriguing side stories. In Chapter IX, we'll suggest answers as to why Uncle Charlie remained a bachelor after several failed attempts at close companionship. You'll be left to decide which reasons make sense to you. Best of all, you may find some centenarian wisdom for yourself.

Foreword: Sally

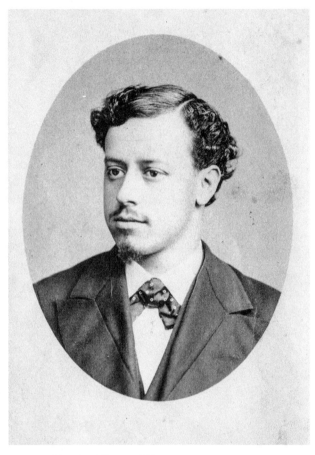

Charles Wesley Thiery as a young man

What can the people living today learn from Charles Wesley Thiery, AKA Great Uncle Charlie, born in 1850?

I never met Uncle Charlie in person, I know him only through his interviews, photos, and family stories that have been passed down. The spirit of Uncle Charlie lives on and we can benefit from the way he took on life in his time.

Uncle Charlie lived life his way—going against family and societal expectations when he felt he needed to. He stayed single, traveled, changed careers, and remained young in his mind while the years passed on the calendar. Most telling is the fact he worked full time until age 93 and didn't consider himself "old" until age 96. From retirement until his death 14 years later, Uncle Charlie was actively involved in his community. Uncle Charlie's support network (before there was even a word for

THE SOCIAL GENERATIONS, WHICH refer to people more or less living at the same time, have nicknames recognized by demographers. Among the more current ones are the Millennials (born 1980-2000) and Generation X (born 1965-1979). I fall into the Baby Boomers group (born 1946-1964).

it) and his own strong identity maintained him until he reached the finish line at age 107 ½.

The best message I've learned from Uncle Charlie is that having a strong self-image is a very useful trait to be successful in this world. Uncle Charlie was the type who could look in a mirror and know who he was. He would give God the credit, but he himself has to be acknowledged for his demeanor, especially at the advanced age when he was covered in the press. His sharp sense of humor made him a popular subject in the Boston area and beyond for interviews and recognition.

So, the next time you need some inspiration to be strong against the culture of today, think of Uncle Charlie. Looking to Napoleon as his role model, Uncle Charlie was his own man as he faced the inevitable challenges one encounters in a lifetime. Know Uncle Charlie is with us (in the next world) as we strive to live long and live well in this one.

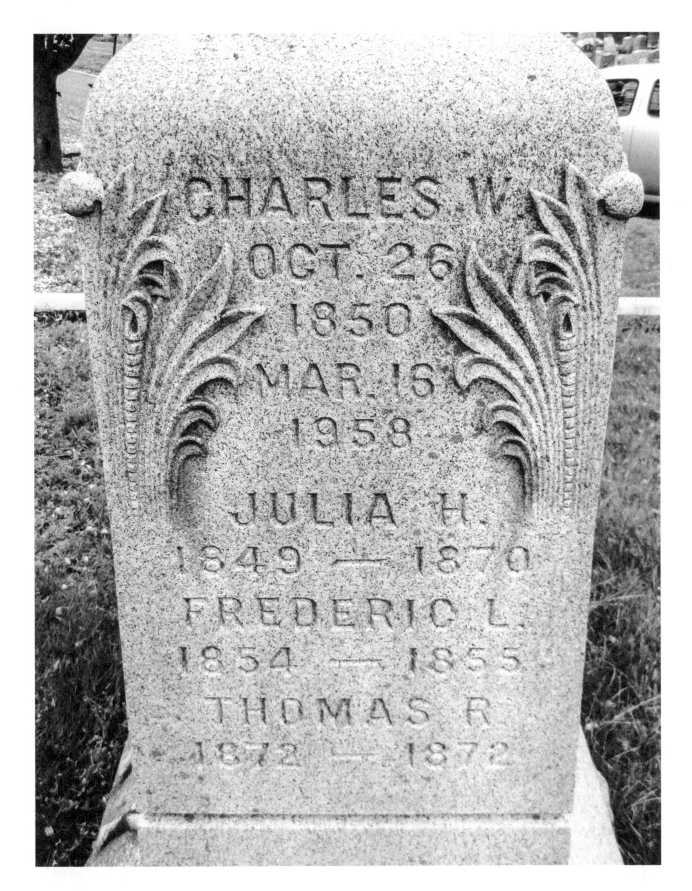

Chapter 1.

"The strong die before the weak."

CENTENARIAN WISDOM

OCTOBER 26TH, 1850, CHARLES Wesley Thiery, AKA my Great Uncle Charlie, was born in Cambridge, Massachusetts. The average man born back then wouldn't make it beyond 38. Saturday, October 26th, 1957, the North Adams Massachusetts Transcript announced "Belmont, MA, Charles Wesley Thiery, who almost died of pneumonia when he was two, is 107 today. A spry thin, little man (5'3"), he has white whiskers, a quick step, and a firm handclasp." As a child, I often sat and talked with Uncle Charlie. I loved hearing about his life. His opinions were insightful and often with tongue in cheek.

On March 16, 1958, the old man's friend, pneumonia, took Uncle Charlie.

Uncle Charlie made many light-hearted quips. When he was asked what his formula was for a long life, our family often heard, "I don't drink or smoke. I have no children to worry me and no wife to scold me!" He repeated the same thing to many news reporters and, on occasion, "I'm a Lifelong Republican". He once said he had no special "theory" for long life. Really! The truth: he had seven healthy habits and a mindset to survive into his 108th year.

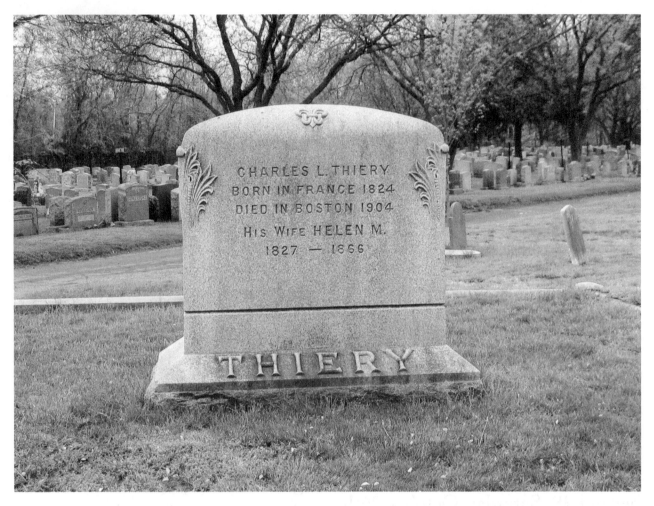

By Uncle Charlie's account, he was a "mischievous youngster" until age 15 when he lost his mother to Bright's disease (a urinary track illness). In that same year, at a revival at his Harvard Street Methodist church, he committed to Christianity. He continued active church membership until his death—ninety-two years later.

Five years later, his sister, Julia, also died of Bright's disease. She was 21. I, too, lost a parent at 15, my father, John Thiery Batchelder. It took me fifteen years to feel secure again. However, my spiritual life has developed over decades, it was not an epiphany.

Did Uncle Charlie ever get over the death of his mother? Did it influence him to remain a bachelor?

One of Uncle Charlie's more serious statements was, "The strong die before the weak." He claimed that he had to watch his diet because of stomach trouble that he had throughout his life. In one news story, he said his stomach trouble began when he "came in from the outside" to work in his father's business. He exclaimed, "Father's business was in a precarious state." At age 100, it was reported, "Thiery says he never has been very well." On his 106th birthday he told one reporter, "I've always had to watch what I ate…and take good care of myself." Chapter III covers Dr. White, President Eisenhower's cardiologist, who wrote extensively about Uncle Charlie's health history, including his medical exam findings.

Beginning at age 22, I had frequent physical exams required for Air Force flying duty. They continued for three decades. These exams built the habit of monitoring my health. Next, our air crew aviation physiology training taught us the hazards of smoking and drinking. Cigarettes and alcohol kill the oxygen carrying capacity of the blood to the brain. Inhaling the smoke of two cigarettes effectively places one at 5,000 feet altitude—less oxygen. Therefore, if you're flying at 5,000 feet, physiologically you are at 10,000 feet and require supplemental oxygen. If aircrew members are getting inadequate amounts of sleep, they will lose their ability to be effective aviators. During sleep, the body re-energizes itself. "Eight hours from bottle to throttle!" was the rule. This refers to the time it takes to clear alcohol from our system.

In Uncle Charlie's later years he had a heart attack. He commented on how he was careful to manage himself by not overdoing it. He seemed to sense the activity that put him at risk and adjust. For example, at his home at 121 Hammond Road, if out of breath from climbing the series of steps to his second floor apartment, he would stop at the landings to rest.

He didn't walk his usual mile or two if it were raining. Perhaps this is because he feared pneumonia. Boston is well known for cold, clammy wet weather. My personal

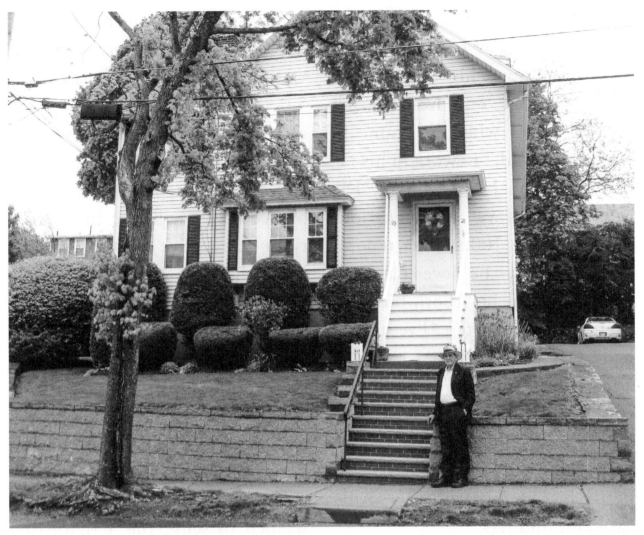

Uncle Charlie's Residence from 1942-1958

memory is how often he was wearing a scarf, and we have many pictures of him in hat, overcoat, and scarf. If he had trouble sleeping because of indigestion, he would sit upright in bed for a few hours. Uncle Charlie was very aware of his body.

Practicing Hatha yoga beginning around age 40, I became more aware of my body. For example, when I was experiencing more stress than usual in business, or personal matters, such as going through a divorce at age 47, I would close the office door, pull out a floor mat, and take 30 minutes or more to relax and re-charge my "batteries." I utilized those exercises that lower the pulse rate and helped me to breathe deeper and get more energy.

The following chapters will illustrate seven of eight healthy habits that Uncle Charlie maintained, allowing him to live over two and half times longer than the average man born in 1850.

Uncle Charlie's Daily Routine at Age 100

7 AM He arose and ate a "hearty breakfast." For up to 2 hours he read newspapers covering local, national, and international news and events. He then made the bed. "I always insisted on making my own bed. I need the exercise."

"Then, I generally sit down for some serious reading, non-fiction preferences…" For example, books about his hero, Napoleon. A reporter noted he had one of the largest collections in the area.

Uncle Charlie would enjoy a complete luncheon; next, he'd generally rest for an hour before walking one to two miles, if it was not raining.

He would return from his afternoon activities and have a light evening meal. After that, he would read some more. He would adjust his schedule for his frequent club meetings and events.

"I get to bed around 9 PM." He got enough rest; I count at least nine hours.

"I enjoy life every minute of every day." Note: I've learned that scripters with heavier pen pressure get more satisfaction out of everyday life. Uncle Charlie's writing strokes showed depth. Heavier down pressure with writing instruments is usually associated with those scripters savoring daily moments more than light line writers. They can relive their memories longer (see Chapter II, 47 Dominate Traits).

Charles Wesley Thiery's formula (September 15, 1953 news report) "I didn't get married; I don't use tobacco or alcohol; I do what the Bible says."

Josh's Daily Routine

Single people have far greater opportunity to set and maintain their daily habits. Mine were far simpler to manage when I was single for a

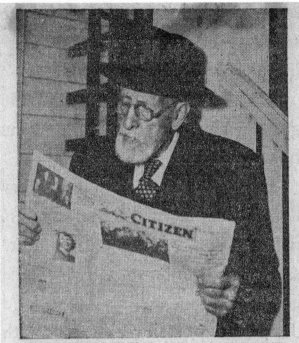

TO BE 104 NEXT TUESDAY — Approaching his 104th birthday, which he will observe next Tuesday, Oct. 26, Belmont's amazing Charles Wesley Thiery keeps abreast of town happenings by scanning the Citizen with his still keen eyes on the steps of his home at 121 Hammond rd.

Mr. Thiery, a bachelor and a retired gold refiner, was born and lived most of his life in Cambridge before coming to Belmont eleven years ago to make his home with Mr. and Mrs. L. Frank Merrick. He is frequently seen striding through Cushing Square and when he has business in Boston hops aboard an MTA car.

He is the unchallenged oldest member of the Republican Club of Massachusetts and has been a member of the Harvard-Epworth Methodist Church of Cambridge for eighty-seven years.
(Hird photo)

number of years. Currently, by necessity, I need flexibility. In order to limit stress, I must adjust to interruptions and changes. I cannot obsess over missing scheduled activities. I set goals. For example, I strive for thirty minutes of recumbent bike cycling seven days a week. To avoid boredom, I read, watch TV, or listen to ballgames on the radio. I can live with a minimum of four sessions per week. I plan Hatha yoga exercises for seven times per week; five is acceptable. Still in business at 83, and having a wife, four children, seven grandchildren, plus active memberships in business associations and Kiwanis requires schedule changes and adjusting for priorities. Complicating matters, Betty Ann Sage, my wife, has three children, five grandchildren, and one great granddaughter. Sharing our home is a little black miniature schnauzer, Kelly. So, you can imagine the family demands.

Between 5 to 6 AM, I rise and eat breakfast. Usually it consists of herbal tea (sweetened with stevia) and fresh fruit. I understand it's best to have fruit by itself before or after meals. 30 minutes later I will have my buttered toast with sugar free preserves. Ideally, waking up and enjoying breakfast is not rushed. Should you start your day with stress, you will be burned out before the day is over.

Like Uncle Charlie, I read the local, national, and international news at breakfast. I make our king sized bed. Yes, I've learned from

Uncle Charlie that it is exercise! My business day begins around 7 AM, writing, phoning, and coordinating activities with associates until 11:30. Lunch is with associates, spouse, clients, or at business meetings, usually ending at 12:30 or 1 PM. My business efforts continue on until around 3:30 PM, when I usually attempt to have a 75 minute nap. After a nap, I retrieve and respond to new messages. Then it's time for hatha yoga exercise and passive mediation. Dinner begins between 5:30 and 6:30 PM. After supper, there are local chores—domestic stuff, shopping, etc. Around 7:30 to 8 PM I begin my 30 minutes of recumbent cycling, reading to avoid boredom. Between 9 to 9:30 PM, Betty Ann and I begin letting go of the day by playing Spite and Malice. While playing this card game, we switch the TV channels between Fox News and ballgames, etc. If Uncle Charlie were here today, he would be a Fox News fan.

10:45 PM Shower. Bedtime around 11 PM.

My average total sleep time, including afternoon naps, is about seven hours. There are interruptions. For example, phone calls from children and grandchildren and play time with Kelly, who will jump onto our laps whenever it suits her. All of these needs can result in getting less rest than ideal. Local and cross country business travel interferes with sleep as well. This is where hatha yoga deep breathing exercises allows one to rebuild their energy for the remaining hours of the day. My Bible study group meets at 7:15 AM on Thursdays. It can get passed over due to local business associations' responsibilities. Thankfully, Saturdays and Sundays lighten up with only three to four hours of business activity, including investment property management. From navigating and piloting for over thirty years with the Air Force and the Civil Air Patrol, I learned the necessity of being flexible. If I wasn't flexible, adjusting to the unexpected changes to flight, business, and family plans, I'd really be stressed. As a single man, Uncle

Charlie controlled his stress by being very decisive. Chapter X, Uncle Charlie's words, "I closed the door on many I didn't agree with." He didn't get resentful waiting for others to show up for appointments. I remember one time when my father didn't drive up at the 9 AM appointed hour for their annual Memorial Day trip to the cemetery. Uncle Charlie returned to his second story quarters that year; thereafter, my father was on time. Uncle Charlie's message was clear: He did not wait on people, even family. In a newspaper interview headlined "Oldest Republican", asked how to avoid stress Uncle Charlie replied, "I'm not much for fretting about anything either."

Being an author, to complete this eighth book, required sequestering myself and depending upon an understanding spouse; and, counting on a tolerant co-author. If all else fails, remember gerontologist Dr. William Osler's advice: "Get a chronic disease and take good care of it."

Chapter 2.

"He liked his free time when he could find it..."

FORTY-SEVEN DOMINANT TRAITS OF THE LEGEND

BEGINNING IN 1999, FOR four major cruise ship lines, I've had fun entertaining on-board audiences with handwriting analysis. For simplicity's sake, I focus on the dominant personality traits of volunteered writing samples which are an intensity rating of 4 or more on a scale of 0 to 10. For three minutes or so, my laser pointing identifies the source of each trait in the writing strokes, the slant, margins, spacing and other aspects. In Chapter XI, to evaluate Uncle Charlie's behavior, Eileen Page puts all the traits together in meaningful clusters. By then, you will have become familiar with Uncle Charlie through his many statements and facts about his life, to appreciate Eileen's evaluation of his personality shown in his handwriting. That may allow you to ponder reasons why he remained a bachelor.

From the thousands of subject writing samples I've observed since 1976, I don't believe I've seen a sub-

Nov. 14, 1956

Dear Nancy,

I did not feel in any condition to write, nor do I feel in any condition for any thing. Perhaps you will be able to understand it when you reach the age of 106. But I must write or I will not get any letters from you and that would be too bad for I remember I was reading of you traveling in Europe, Asia and Africa and of course I desire to receive, or hear about it all from you. But I am sure that you will want to learn some thing of our recent election, that kind that is of a personal nature. Well, my birth day had some attraction. The Governor & the President sent me congratulation, the President adding words of his own. This I shall keep for future generation to read.

Yesterday I received a letter from Charlie — which was a newspaper article about me. They are interesting of course all because I passed the century mark. Most of these were telegrams. The fact of your traveling so like yours. It especially interests me as to how your

ject with more dominant traits than Uncle Charlie presents in his handwriting. His heavy writing strokes/pressure signifies persistent emotional memory. I know that his depth-of-feeling was strong and allowed him to enjoy reliving his experiences; he "enjoyed every moment of every day." This trait is compounded by the magnification of all his traits from his very small writing stokes—indicating concentration. He was so much into living-in-the-moment that he didn't think about his age until at a birthday party given by his Odd Fellows Club when they gave him a bouquet of 96 roses. Uncle Charlie said, "I didn't make very much over it. I thanked them for it and returned to my seat. It wasn't until those roses opened out, full bloom, at home, and I looked at them and thought—each one of these stands for 365 days of 24 hours each—that I realized for the first time I was an old man."

I too, was so into living, flying for the Air Force, that I didn't stop to shoot all the great camera scenes I could have captured.

The 14 November 1956 source letter was written to my sister, Nancy, at the time in the Foreign Service in South Africa, about two and one half years after Uncle Charlie had an awkward personal encounter with her. All of his dominant traits are clearly presented.

It is exciting to use handwriting analysis to look back and better understand family members and others who have come before us.

Analytical: Sharp V shaped strokes that reach the baseline. Uncle Charlie checked everything out before he tried something new.

Attention, desiring: Final stroke on word ending high and bending back.

Attention Span, Long: Tiny, lower case strokes, very small. This trait would facilitate concentrated reading or work. Uncle Charlie was a voracious reader.

Argumentative: Long lead in stroke.

Broadminded: Broad a's and o's

Caution: A long initial stroke. Uncle Charlie combined this trait with be-

cash the same, surely you do not pay for the same. You must make it business for the Government.

Thanksgiving comes next week and I expect to dine with Janie & her mate (and baby) They have built a house in Bedford. I have seen it in the rough and expect to see it greatly changed when I see next Thursday. The Gov't has a flying field in Bedford, I saw it about two years ago. It would be a nice place to live but it too far from Boston for one who has lived so near to Boston as many years as I have.

My last letter to you was sent from Boston Post Office by air mail I supposed you received it. The Post Office stamp agent told me to put it in an elevated receptical & I suppose you received it, think it was about four months ago (4) Next week is Thanksgiving and soon after will be Christmas, the interesting part of the year. Our summer was all that we could ask for and now we await the winter. The little cold we have had so far I I did not like so I am looking forward to a near future I don't want so you can imagine how I view our near future. But I will be thinking of you basking in African sunshine & waiting your next letter. With kindest regards from
your Uncle Charlie

ing analytical; you'd understand him being slow before he jumped into anything new.

Clannish: Small loop at the end below baseline on y, g or j.

Cultured: Greek E or figure 8 strokes.

Decisive: He was strongly so, except when facing dilemmas. Short or abbreviated word ending strokes.

Dignity: Retraced d and t-stems.

Details: Medium attention to details. The distance of i-dots above his stems and no omitted t-bars both indicate attention to details. Often, when folks get older, they become less likely to enjoy dealing with excessive details.

Determination: Very strong—extended straight y down-strokes.

Direct: Elimination of unnecessary beginning up-strokes. He was most often very direct and outspoken. Otherwise he could be indecisive.

Dominate/dictatorial/domineering: Sharply down slanted t-bars.

Emotional Memory: Strong pen downward pressure indicates very long lasting.

Exploratory: Saw tooth, pointed tops in h, m or n.

Factual: Straight y down-strokes below his baseline, without loops.

Fatalistic: Example, the return of the down stroke of y crosses before the baseline and falls over.

Fluidity: Strokes flowing from one letter to the next. For example, often in the beginning letters of a word the ending stroke goes into the next letter, for example with W or H. Dr. Paul Dudley White had very fluid handwriting, see Chapter III, Dr. White's letter to Mr. Ross.

Frank: Clear lower case o and a.

Goals: Next year or so, understandable in light of his age. t-bars midrange above lower case letter tops.

Generosity: Generosity is shown in handwriting by broad word ending up-strokes without countering traits, such as squeezed letters or ending stroke hooks. Though Uncle

Charlie could be very generous, he gave gifts based on his values and opinions.

Hesitation: Very long lead in strokes. Notice in his letters he still refers to his indiscretion with sister Nancy (Chapter IX); he's reliving it.

Humor: Concave, upper zone, flowing lead in strokes often seen on W and H.

Impatient: i-dots jump beyond i-stems, rightward is the future. Also t-bars to the right of stem, or just touching the stem.

Indecisive: Extended straight ending strokes. When unresolved issues or new questions arose, Uncle Charlie was indecisive.

Intuition: Breaks between letters in words, after second letter.

Investigative: Inverted like ^ on m and n. Sharper, not rounded.

Irritability: Flicks in lieu of rounded i-dots. This can be seen in Uncle Charlie's writing when referring to his and Nancy's graveside visit.

Loner: Straight y down-stokes without loops. Uncle Charlie had his private side.

Manual Dexterity: Note the precision clearness in his well-formed writing, even in his smaller strokes. Amazing for a centenarian.

Obstinate: Variable. Stiff t-stem legs. Still, he was often able to bend (t-legs bending).

Optimistic: Baseline slant upward. Clearly indicated.

Patient: Rounded i-dots directed above i-stems. Generally, but can lose it when he refers to something he can't control, such as when Mrs. Merritt (landlady) was in the hospital.

Perseverance: Extra-long straight down-strokes, below the baseline, seen in lower case y's and g's.

Philosophical Interests: Lower case l and h strokes well above the middle zone.

Physically minded: Lower case p-loops.

Precise: Short/balanced t-bars, retraced p-stems.

Pride: t and d-stems two and one half times the height of lower case letters.

Procrastination: t-bars ending at t-stems.

Protective/traditional: He was very protective/traditional of his family name. Notice, in his will, the arcade stroke over the Thiery family name (Chapter IV).

Responsive: Rightward slanted up-strokes. He could empathize with others' problems. He generously helped relatives in need if their values didn't offend him.

Rigid: Straight baselines.

Sensory perception: The depth and pressure of writing heavier or lighter.

Stubborn: Stiff t and d-stem legs. Variable, he could bend sometimes.

Vanity: t or d-stems over three times the high of lower case letters. Uncle Charlie's pride at times bordered on vanity.

Variety: Large lower loops. He fulfilled his need for change from all the organizations he belonged to, his extensive reading, and networking with contacts in his sales career.

Willpower: Heavy stroke t-bars. Longer t-bars equal longer application of will power.

Signature: Your signature is a reflection of what you want the world to know about you. The given name reveals how you feel about yourself, in comparison to how you feel about your family or husband's name. An Illegible signature suggests the writer may be trying to hide something, especially one that is encircled. An easily read signature, clear and open, that's congruent with the body of writing, means what you see is what you get. Uncle Charlie's signature in his letter to Nancy, found in Chapter IX, was authentic. However, the signature in his will was different from his signature when writing a loved one. Uncle Charlie was very protective of the family name.

Chapter 3.
"The Heart of a Boy"
A MEDICAL MARVEL

EISENHOWER'S CARDIOLOGIST
PAUL DUDLEY WHITE, MD,
REPORTS

I remember well my immediate family talk about Uncle Charlie: No signs of hardening of the arteries until he was well into his 90s. In all our visits I experienced a hale, hearty, and enthusiastic man. Often I'd heard of his daily walks of a mile or two. This practice is a great stress reducer. Remember, Uncle Charlie's decisive return to his apartment when my father failed to pick him up on time for an appointment. With my maturing, I understand that as good stress reduction behavior. He avoided resentment by acting decisively. No fuming or fussing.

In another news story, Uncle Charlie "believes his pneumonia at age 2½ shrunk his bellows (lungs), so that several times he almost drowned swimming in the Charles River near his boyhood home. It also gave him a mild attack of St. Vitus dance." Sydenham's chorea or chorea minor (historically referred to as Saint Vitus Dance) is a disorder characterized by rapid, uncoordinated jerking movements, primarily affecting the face, hands, and feet. "Thiery says he never has been very well."

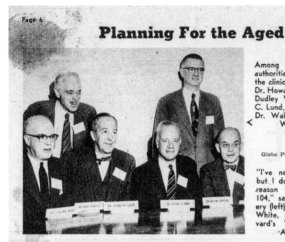

Planning For the Aged

Among the world-famous authorities who attended the clinic were (left to right) Dr. Howard F. Root, Dr. Paul Dudley White, Dr. Charles C. Lund, Dr. Dean A. Clark, Dr. Walter E. Barton, Dr. Walter Bauer.

Globe Photos • Gil Friedberg

"I've never been married, but I don't think that's the reason I'm so healthy at 104," says Charles W. Thiery (left) to Dr. Paul Dudley White, a speaker at Harvard's "Problems of the Aging" clinic.

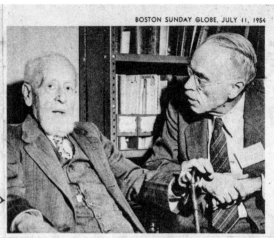

BOSTON SUNDAY GLOBE, JULY 11, 1954

RIGHT PHOTO: Charles Wesley Thiery, left, Dr. Paul Dudley White, right

But let's look to the eminent cardiologist Paul Dudley White for a medical report about Uncle Charlie. Dr. White pioneered advancing the critical importance of exercise for recovery of illnesses, accidents, and the part it plays in extending longevity. Dr. White's famous quotes include, "A vigorous five-mile walk will do more good for an unhappy but otherwise healthy adult than all the medicine and psychology in the world." "Walk more, eat less, sleep more." "I wish we could do something useful with tobacco—like making fertilizer out of it." Wikipedia states: "Dr. White was a prominent advocate of preventative medicine…his first scientific paper, co-authored with Dr. Roger Lee, was about measuring the speed of blood coagulation (1913). This methodology is still in use today."

Atlanta doctor, Allan C. Bleich, MD, board certified in internal medicine, met with Dr. White years ago. He said Dr. White was likely the first to recognize the importance of regular exercise for extending longevity.

Josh's reflections

Dr. White presented Uncle Charlie as having the "heart of a boy"; and, writing in a letter to Mr. Ross, October 24, 1954, said, "I consider Mr. Thiery to be my prize patient, although he is so healthy that he

Sunday,
October 24, 1954.

Dear Mr. Ross,

I am writing to ask you to tell Mr. Thiery and your president how greatly I regret my inability to be present on Tuesday evening to help to honor Mr. Thiery's 104th birthday because of a very important prior engagement. I regret this exceedingly, especially since I consider Mr. Thiery to be my prize patient although I would add that he is so healthy that he can hardly be called a patient. May I call him instead a very warm friend.

Mr. Thiery during the last four years has helped me immeasurably

33

in my teaching, by the demonstration
of his physical and mental alertness
despite pneumonia which nearly
killed him 102 years ago, nervous
indigestion all his life, 82 years of
hard work (he retired at 93), and
bundle branch block by electrocardio-
gram.

Best wishes to Mr. Charles
Thiery and to you all. I hope
that I may be invited to attend
his 105th birthday a year from
now.

Sincerely Yours,

Paul E. White, M.D.

can hardly be called a patient." One of Dr. White's specialties was preventive medicine. Uncle Charlie proved that he himself was a master of preventive medicine. He listened to his body, he analyzed his symptoms, and he adjusted his lifestyle.

More comments from news stories are helpful to prove this last point.

"Mr. Thiery suffered a brief spell of rheumatism during his 80's and doesn't care to risk a reoccurrence, so he takes a brisk walk about the neighborhood, a mile or more daily. 'I've got plenty of time and suffered a heart attack some years back. I climb up the stairs very slowly, resting on each landing.'"

I conclude that Uncle Charlie succeeded very well, considering all of his reported statements which include: "The strong die before the weak." "I had to watch my diet because I had stomach trouble throughout my life." Note: Uncle Charlie often sat up in bed to alleviate his indigestion.

One newspaper article noted Uncle Charlie's regular physician (not Dr. White) predicted he would die within one year of retiring. Uncle Charlie retired at age 93 when the limited gold supply made working in his field unprofitable. That same reporter noted, "so he devoted himself to keeping busy reading his books, which are stacked up everywhere in his room."

Uncle Charlie's focus was on seven of our eight healthy habits. He recognized his weaknesses and compensated. By the time you finish reading this book, I hope you appreciate how Uncle Charlie's life exemplifies applied preventative medicine, and you will use his centenarian wisdom, too.

CHARLES W. THIERY: 1850 TO 1958

By PAUL D. WHITE, M.D.

BOSTON, MASS.

What are the reasons for survival and good health in centenarians? It is probably just as important to try to obtain correct answers to this question as it is to solve the mysteries of death from disease in early life or in middle age.

Born of Huguenot stock in Cambridge, Massachusetts, on October 26th, 1850, Charles Thiery was almost fatally ill with pneumonia at the age of two but survived more than 105 years longer before he did finally succumb to bronchopneumonia on March 16, 1958. In childhood besides the usual children's diseases he had chorea and scarlet fever, and he broke his arm when he fell from a tree. At the age of 20 years he had "slow" (? typhoid) fever but after that he had very little illness until his final pneumonia. There were occasional colds or attacks of grippe, one of which was rather severe in his 104th year and required a good many weeks of convalescence. He also for many years was bothered somewhat by "nervous indigestion" which, he said, prevented him from eating as much as most of his friends who died at much younger ages. His only other complaint was that he was somewhat hard of hearing which, however, was not very evident most of the time following my first examination of him three days after his 100th birthday.

Mr. Thiery was always a very active man, walking long distances in his youth—at one time he walked 25 miles in 5 hours—and riding a horse, especially when he was in military service in the cavalry. Even in his old age he continued to walk a lot and averaged a mile or more a day during the last few years of his life. He was always very spry when I used to go to the house where he lived to take him to my office or to hospital clinics for examination and presentation to my graduate students or to medical society meetings about twice a year from 1950 on. There was a rather long and steep flight of steps leading from his front door to the sidewalk and he regularly scorned my proffered arm and tripped down the flight like a healthy man half his age.

Mr. Thiery never married but on occasion said that he didn't believe

It is a pleasure to express my appreciation to Dr. Walter Feeley, Mr. Thiery's family physician, Dr. Raymond Thiery, Charles Thiery's nephew, Mrs. Nathaniel Tufts, his niece, and Dr. R. Stenger, pathologist at the Massachusetts General Hospital, for their help in preparing this report.

152

that his bachelorhood was responsible for his great longevity. Neither did he smoke nor drink but he did think that his long life was favored by his avoidance of tobacco and alcohol. He ate well but sparingly and was never obese. He didn't like eggs but he did eat a good deal of ice cream and liked butter, milk, cream, and pastry. His indigestion, mentioned above, never took a severe form and he was never thought by his medical advisors to suffer from a peptic ulcer. He enjoyed life, liked company, and spoke easily and wittily with a cheerful twinkle in his eye. He kept up with the news, both local and worldwide, and enjoyed the annual birthday parties which were arranged for him by his friends and various social groups. He had met the President after he himself had reached an advanced age and sent his greetings and best wishes to him by way of my own visits to Denver during the President's illness in the fall of 1955—in fact they exchanged birthday congratulations at that time. Occasionally Mr. Thiery would reminisce, for example, about the American Civil War which began when he was 11 and ended when he was 15. Lincoln and Grant were great heroes of his, as were later Theodore Roosevelt and Dwight Eisenhower; in fact he voted for Grant for President when he reached voting age.

Mr. Thiery started his first job in silver and gold-smithing under his father's tutelage at 11 years and retired at the age of 93, 82 years later. He fitted in some schooling on the side, however, in his youth and was a well read man. He travelled little but followed the news of the world with avid interest.

His family history was important and it was quite obvious that heredity was on his side despite the fact that his mother died of "Bright's disease" at the age of 39 and a sister of the "same disease" at 21. His father died at 79, a brother at 92, and a second sister at 85. He did not know about his grandparents.

Physical examination by myself on October 29th, 1950, three days after his hundredth birthday, revealed a healthy appearing elderly man with white hair, beard, and mustache, short (63 inches) and slight (115 pounds) in build, a little hard of hearing but with no other complaints. He submitted to the examination at the request of a friend of his who was a patient of mine. His eyesight was good with normal pupils and no arcus senilis. There was no abnormal pulse in the neck. The heart was normal in size and sounds, the second doubled at the base. There were no murmurs. There were occasional premature beats at a rate of 68. The blood pressure measured 140 mm. systolic and 70 mm. diastolic. There was no evidence of congestive failure. There was a palpable arterial pulse in the ankles. There was moderate scoliosis but very little kyphosis.

Fluoroscopic examination by myself showed a full but apparently normal sized heart with dense but not dilated aorta; the lung fields were clear.

A few years later orthodiagraphic measurements were as follows: the transverse diameter of the heart 10.8 cm. and the internal diameter of the thorax 24.2 cm.

The electrocardiogram at the time of my examination three days after his 100th birthday was the first that he had ever had taken. It showed occasional ventricular premature beats, one of which was interpolated, at a rate of 70 to 80, averaging 75, and left bundle branch block; the P-R interval was normal. Annual electrocardiograms during the next seven years showed little or no change; the last one taken on December 10th, 1957, three months before he died, showed normal rhythm without premature beats but still with bundle branch block, at a rate of 65 to 70.

Annually and sometimes semiannually it was my privilege to examine and often to demonstrate Mr. Thiery at teaching clinics and at medical society meetings. His cooperation at such times was more than generous and his mental acuity, wit, and memory of historic events during the last century, such as the American Civil War, added color to the clinical exercises. The last of the larger audiences before which he appeared was the American College of Physicians at their annual meeting in Boston in the spring of 1957, a year before his death. My notes on his record that day were as follows:

April 11, 1957. Shown at special clinic at the Massachusetts General Hospital for the American College of Physicians. Has been very well all summer, fall, and winter, averaging a mile or more a day walking in Belmont. The only trouble has been an accident three days ago when he was dragged on the road for a few yards when his coat got caught in the door of a taxi as he alighted. The only injury was a bruise on the hand.

Physical examination: Alert. Pulse regular at 72. Blood pressure 148 mm. systolic and 75 diastolic. Heart—good sounds, grade ½ precordial systolic murmur.

Fluoroscopy: Normal (full) heart size. Aorta slightly dense. Lungs clear. Moderate scoliosis.

Electrocardiogram: Normal rhythm, rate 75, left bundle branch block.

Comment: In excellent health.

Rx. Reassurance. Carry on as now. To see in 6 or 8 months.

During the seven years of my contact with Mr. Thiery prior to his death he was only once really ill. That was in the winter of 1953 to 1954, when as already mentioned, he had a prolonged respiratory infection. During his long convalescence he developed considerable soft pitting edema of both legs equally to his knees and ruefully he suggested that his end was approaching. However, since his heart was still normal in size, his neck veins were not engorged, and he had no dyspnea, we believed that the edema was due to local stasis from the effect of gravity; he had spent day after day sitting in a chair. Also there was no evidence of phlebitis.

Therefore, he was advised to begin to walk again, which he did daily and within a fortnight the edema had entirely cleared and never returned.

Mr. Thiery was always alert in appearance with a kind expression and his handwriting remained clear and steady to the end. One of his letters to me which he sent early in 1951 was of particular interest with respect to his diet and indigestion. I shall quote it herewith in full:

Feb. 1, 1951. Dear doctor:

Answering yours of Jan. 29 will say that the matter of my diet is a very important one to me and has been from my infancy. It showed up at first when I was 3 days old and has continued until now. When 3 days old I demanded something to *eat* so I started with 2½ seed-cakes soaked in milk and as a boy was always a hearty eater and as a boy always, if possible, out of doors. The heartiest food was what I craved and this continued until after working indoors for years I found lighter food suited me more. Later, taking on responsibility, the strain affected my nervous system and I began to have attacks of indigestion of which I have had many for years back, all of which were of a frightful nature. The last one occurred about 4 years ago and the usual faint turned to a convulsion. The cause—stewed corn not properly chewed.

For nearly a year I have had some cream with my crackers and milk for my supper two thirds of the week and bread and butter with perhaps a little cake. Eggs I don't eat in any form unless in something already cooked. They do not agree with me. Butter seems all right.

I have to be careful about going up stairs after dinner, or my heart is affected. In the middle of the day I can eat a fair sized dinner with other people.

If I eat a fairly good meal, as above, just before retiring, I use my back rest to sit up the first quarter of the night, and lie down the rest of the night. I am not a good sleeper generally. I seldom go out of an evening.

My strange start in life was because my parents were poor but honest and my mother lived mostly on brown bread until she gagged, so she said.

Hope this will answer your inquiry. Charles W. Thiery.

Finally, early in March of 1958, Mr. Thiery's landlord, Mr. Merrick, who was in his 90's, fell and after a few days died, followed very shortly by the death of Mr. Merrick's wife who had been very frail for years and was also of a very advanced age. During this upset of the household Mr. Thiery also fell trying to help and very shortly afterwards was found to have pneumonia. He was taken to a nursing home and treated with antibiotics and nursing care but succumbed to his illness a week later on March 16th. Immediate permission for a postmortem examination was granted by the three nephews and one niece of Mr. Thiery. This revealed the following: bronchopneumonia, bilateral, in the lower lobes (undoubtedly the immediate cause of death), moderate bilateral pulmonary emphysema, moderate coronary atherosclerosis with an old recanalized (and symptomless) occlusion of the right coronary atrery, marked atherosclerosis of the aorta, cholelithiasis (which may have played a role in his "indigestion"), benign nephrosclerosis, benign prostatic hypertrophy, and senile atrophy of the liver. The heart weighed 400 grams.

DISCUSSION

There is little to add to this account in the way of discussion. Every centenarian is asked why he lived so long. Usually the answer is "by the grace of God" which was also one of Mr. Thiery's several answers. Such a reason is, of course, a combination of the influence of heredity, an escape from serious accidents and fatal infections, and the effect of the ways of life. Doubtless all three of these factors were operative in Mr. Thiery's case—we cannot credit any one for the entire responsibility nor even more can we credit any one item in any of the three causes, for example, his abstinence from the use of tobacco or alcohol or the fact that he never married, or even his nervous indigestion which prevented him from eating as much as some of his friends who died a generation earlier. Doubtless his slight body build was an advantage as has been shown in the case of experimental animals. His program of regular exercise maintained throughout life was in all probability helpful. Neither infections of which he had his share nor his nervous sensitivity which was of rather high degree, shortened his life until he had his final pneumonia which used to be called the old man's friend, not necessarily applicable in his case since had he survived he might have lived another few years in good health, as I had found him when I examined him last three months before he died.

Two other points should be emphasized. His bundle branch block discovered at the time of his first electrocardiogram at the age of one hundred years and three days was only of passing interest; it certainly did not shorten his life and it may have been present for a good many years before his first electrocardiogram was taken. Secondly, he had neither coronary nor myocardial insufficiency despite a moderate amount of coronary atherosclerosis and one old occlusion. His normal heart size and normal blood pressure were in his favor. His premature beats were unimportant; he never had any serious arrhythmias.

SUMMARY

A brief biography of Charles W. Thiery of Cambridge and Belmont who died recently at the age of 107½ years is herewith presented with particular reference to his health through his long life. It is probable that familial longevity, slight body build, the habit of regular exercise, and a philosophical attitude toward life contributed to his longevity. He himself also thought that abstinence from tobacco and alcohol was helpful and that his long standing nervous indigestion might have acted favorably to keep down any tendency to overeat. He weathered many infections until his final bronchopneumonia which occurred 105 years after a near-fatal attack of pneumonia in early childhood.

DISCUSSION

Dr. Frederick T. Billings Jr. (Nashville): Dr. White, we obviously rarely get an opportunity to participate in such a study in the life of a gentleman of this age, and those of us, who lead the busy life of a doctor, have heard, untruthfully, that doctors lead short lives. We know this is not the case.

You mentioned that he had a philosophical attitude toward life. I wonder what occupation he pursued for the first, say, 70 years of his life, perhaps? I didn't hear you mention his profession.

Dr. White: I forgot to speak of that. He started working when he was 11 years old and retired at 93—thus he worked for 82 years as a silversmith. His father was a silversmith, and in those years, apparently, it was not rare for the father to initiate the son early into his own employment. He got some education on the side and was quite a well read man. He felt that he didn't want to stop working at 93, but circumstances obliged him to do that. He could have carried on so far as his health was concerned.

Dr. Thornton Scott (Lexington): I should like to ask Dr. White for a few details about the man's dietary habits and food preferences. I was reminded of an amusing incident two or three years ago. My father and I were in Chicago at a medical meeting and happened to have breakfast with Dr. Howard Sprague. At that time, the specter of cholesterol was at its most ghastly height, and my father, who was in his eighties and is actively engaged in the practice of medicine, began to attribute his longevity to the fact he had never touched an egg in his life and never touched a drop of milk. Howard Sprague said he had just come from seeing Harvard's oldest living graduate, and he estimated that he had eaten 50,000 eggs.

Dr. White: Mr. Thiery said that he didn't like eggs. He liked butter and ate ice cream quite frequently. He said that he began to eat rather heartily in infancy—and I have a letter which he wrote to me in 1951 about his early diet, he said, "When three days old, I demanded something to eat, so I started with 2½ seed cakes soaked in milk, and as a boy was always a hearty eater and always out of doors. The heartiest food was always what I craved. This continued for years. Later, having taken on responsibility, the strain affected my nervous system, and I began to have attacks of indigestion." He thought that stewed corn not properly chewed was the cause. He ate, I would say, a fairly average American diet except for eggs.

Dr. Edward Rose (Philadelphia): In view of the fact that we are all highly sensitized to the importance and value of necropsy, I wonder who signed his autopsy permit.

Dr. White: I might say that Dr. Castleman's department at the Massachusetts General Hospital did his autopsy, and I believe that his family physician signed his death certificate. Old age doesn't kill a person. It may doubtless make a person more susceptible to strains. My idea is that a person doesn't die of old age. He has either pneumonia or something like it. That reminds me of a record of a woman who died at the age of 45 years in the Massachusetts General Hospital a century ago; her final diagnosis, without any question mark, was "old age." That was in 1856.

Dr. Morton Hamburger (Cincinnati): Perhaps, it is germane to call the attention of the society to a contemporary of Mr. Thiery, Dr. Senner, a distinguished neurologist, who died in Cincinnati last year at 104. There was, apparently, one habit of life in common between the two. Dr. Senner was fond of walking. He was politically more independent than Mr. Thiery. During the campaign of 1952, someone asked him if he was planning to vote for Eisenhower, and he said, "Well, I don't believe I will, because I voted for a general once, and he didn't turn out so well."

DR. GORHAM: I think you failed to answer Dr. Rose's question as to who signed the autopsy permit.

DR. WHITE: Oh, a niece. All his immediate family had died except for one niece and three nephews. I called them all up and they all gave permission. It was the niece, who lived nearby, who actually signed the permit.

Chapter 4.

"I was a mischievous youngster until age 15."

92 YEARS AS A DEDICATED CHRISTIAN, BEGINNING IN 1866

"I WAS A MISCHIEVOUS youngster, always taking chances…sticking my neck out…and getting into trouble. I used to be disgusted with myself every night until I joined the church, but I had a lot of fun, too." Uncle Charlie told the Boston Globe newspaper that he got the most fun out of life during his boyhood years, before he converted to Christianity at age 15 during a revival meeting at the Harvard Street Methodist Church. Note:

1866 was a difficult year for Uncle Charlie. He lost his mother to Bright's disease. He was active in the Massachusetts State Militia Cavalry and he was out of school working for his father in a declining family business. Did Uncle Charlie have guilt over his mother's demise, and was he feeling the loss of her love? Fifteen is a tough time to lose a parent and grow up in wartime. I experienced the same. My spiritual growth has oc-

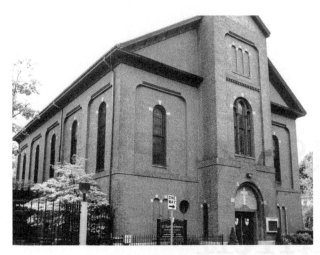

The Harvard Street Methodist Church building where Uncle Charlie converted.

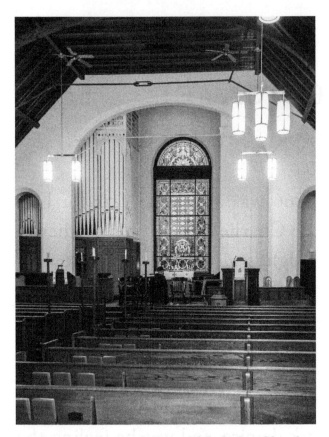

Harvard–Epworth United Methodist Church Sanctuary where Uncle Charlie's 100th birthday service was celebrated.

curred slowly over many years, it's not been an epiphany.

The Harvard Street Methodist Church merged with The Epworth Methodist Church in March of 1941 to form the Harvard-Epworth United Methodist Church. Uncle Charlie continued to worship at the new location, which is located beside the Harvard Law School building.

When Uncle Charlie reached age 100, his beloved church, along with the Wesley Foundation at Harvard University, had a commemorative service in his honor. The program for that event contains a brief biography, and notes that he chose the hymns and sermon topic for the occasion. Chapter V presents Uncle Charlie's will. His bequest to the Harvard-Epworth's endowment fund is growing to this day, and is double the next highest gift. This gift to the church is testimony to the strength of his commitment to deeds in actions.

In my early years I don't recall that I was as "mischievous" as Uncle Charlie was. My only memory

CLASS OF SERVICE		SYMBOLS
This is a full-rate Telegram or Cablegram unless its deferred character is indicated by a suitable symbol above or preceding the address.		DL = Day Letter
		NL = Night Letter
		LC = Deferred Cable
		NLT = Cable Night Letter
		Ship Radiogram

WESTERN UNION

1201

W. P. MARSHALL, PRESIDENT

The filing time shown in the date line on telegrams and day letters is STANDARD TIME at point of origin. Time of receipt is STANDARD TIME at point of destination

1950 OCT

.BA423

B.NWA193 NL PD=NEWTON MASS 21=

CHARLES WESLEY THIERY (BETWEEN 10 AND 1030 AM)=

CARE REV JACKSON BURNS HARVARD EPWORTH METHODIST

CHURCH 1555 MASS AVE CAMBRIDGE MASS=

¶ "A GOOD NAME IS RATHER TO BE CHOSEN THAN GREAT RICHES AND

LOVING FAVOR RATHER THAN SILVER AND GOLD". YOU HAVE CHOSEN THE

BETTER PART. ON THIS AUSPICIOUS ANNIVERSARY, THE CENTENNIAL

OF A WORTHY LIFE ACCEPT MY CONGRATULATIONS AND DEEP AFFECTION=

BISHOP JOHN WESLEY LORD=.

THE COMPANY WILL APPRECIATE SUGGESTIONS FROM ITS PATRONS CONCERNING ITS SERVICE

is playing with matches close to our outside cellar door. It started a small fire that could have been disastrous. My mother was the disciplinarian. There were a few times when I was told to go cut a willow suitable for switching; so, I must have been naughty. The day I told my mother, "Hit me again!" that method of punishment ceased.

Harvard-Epworth Methodist Church

and

Wesley Foundation at Harvard University

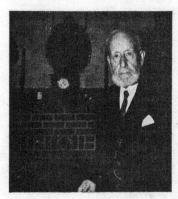

CHARLES WESLEY THIERY, *Our Oldest Member*
One Hundred Years Old, October 26, 1950

JACKSON BURNS, Minister

PAUL STOPENHAGEN, Minister to Students

MRS. R. G. RAMSDELL, Minister's Assistant

RICHARD G. APPEL, Organist

Portions of the church bulletin commemorating Uncle Charlie's 100th Birthday:

Charles Wesley Thiery

It is with deep affection and great pride that we honor today the oldest member of Harvard-Epworth Methodist Church. Mr. Charles Wesley Thiery will be one hundred years old October 26, 1950. He was born on Tremont Street, Cambridge, in 1850.

His father, Charles L. Thiery, was for several years a resident of New York City where he belonged to the John Street Methodist Church. It was in this church that he met the young lady who became his wife. They moved to Boston and later to Cambridge, where he established a watch shop.

Their son, named after the famous Methodist hymn writer, Charles Wesley, attended Webster School, but from time to time was taken out of school to help in his father's shop. His mother died while he was still a boy. He feels that the most important influence in his life has been that of his father. His father's solemn warning that "whatsoever a man soweth that shall he also reap" had an important effect in shaping his life.

Mr. Thiery was converted at a revival service at Harvard Street Methodist Church in 1865. He became a full member of the church in 1866. Soon after he joined he took a Sunday School class of boys. For about thirty years of his life he served as a Sunday School teacher.

In 1875 he went to San Francisco, and transferred his membership to Howard Street Methodist Church in that city. After about a year and a half, however, he returned to Cambridge and to Harvard Street Church. He has been a member of this church (now united with Epworth to form Harvard-Epworth) over eighty-three years.

Mr. Thiery began his business career as a watch case maker and later took up gold refining. His advice to modern business men is: "Always follow the Christian principles . . . On that principle and no other did I do business all my life."

In recent years, Mr. Thiery has lived at 121 Hammond Road, Belmont. He is one of the most faithful attendants at the Sunday services at Harvard-Epworth. His friends unite in wishing him many more years of health and happiness.

The hymns used in the Service today were chosen by Mr. Thiery and he suggested the topic for the sermon. The flowers on the altar are provided by the Official Board as a symbol of appreciation for Mr. Thiery's continuing concern for the welfare of his church.

Order of Worship

Morning Worship, October 22, 1950, at 11:00 o'clock

PRELUDE—"Andante" — Rachmaninoff

INTROIT 60

*HYMN 315—"How Firm a Foundation" — Wade

*CALL TO WORSHIP—

Minister: This is the day which the Lord hath made; let us rejoice and be glad in it.

People: Surely this is none other but the house of God, and this is the gate of heaven.

Minister: Enter into his gates with thanksgiving, and into his courts with praise.

People: The hour cometh, and now is, when the true worshipers shall worship the Father in spirit and in truth.

PRAYER OF CONFESSION

Congregation seated and united in prayer.

Our heavenly Father, who by Thy love hast made us, and through Thy love hast kept us, and in Thy love wouldst make us perfect; we humbly confess that we have not loved Thee with all our heart and soul and mind and strength, and that we have not loved one another as Christ hath loved us. Thy life is within our souls, but our selfishness hath hindered Thee. We have not lived by faith. We have resisted Thy spirit. We have neglected Thine inspirations. Forgive what we have been; help us to amend what we are; and in Thy spirit direct what we shall be; that Thou mayest come into the full glory of Thy creation, in us and in all men, through Jesus Christ our Lord, Amen.

SILENT MEDITATION

WORDS OF ASSURANCE

THE LORD'S PRAYER

**

SCRIPTURE READING Romans 1:8-17

CHORAL RESPONSE (16)

**

ANTHEM—"Brother James Air" — Jacob

PASTORAL PRAYER

CHORAL RESPONSE (596)

**

OFFERTORY—"Jesus, Savior, pilot me" — Schnecker

*DEDICATION OF THE OFFERING (All Uniting) — Number 616

*HYMN 283—"Stand up, stand up for Jesus" — Geibel

SERMON—"I Am Not Ashamed of the Gospel"

*HYMN 287—"A charge to keep I have" — Wesley

*THE BENEDICTION

ORGAN POSTLUDE—"Toccata in F" — Bach

*Congregation Standing   **Ushers may seat late comers

The Wesley Foundation Program

Harvard-Epworth Church has been designated by the Methodist Church as the Wesley Foundation Center for students in the colleges in this vicinity and for local college-age youth.

The regular program of the Foundation includes the following activities:

Sundays—	10:00 A.M.	Wesley Class taught by Prof. Peter Bertocci
	11:00 A.M.	Morning Worship and Sermon
	6:00 P.M.	Fellowship supper (Dine-a-Mite)
	7:00 P.M.	Sanctuary Vesper Service
	7:45 P.M.	Outstanding Speakers, Forums and Discussions (see schedule below)
	9:00 P.M.	Recreation and Refreshments
Wednesdays—	8:00 P.M.	Open House with Discussions, Work Projects and Recreation
Saturdays—		Recreation, Parties, Outings as announced

SUNDAY EVENING PROGRAMS

October 15	THE REVEREND CHARLES PURDHAM "The Church Goes to College"
October 22	STUDENT PANEL "Convictions in Action"
October 29	THE REVEREND JACKSON BURNS "Gandhi's Message for Our Day"
November 5	PROFESSOR HENRY J. CADBURY Harvard University "A Growing Faith"
November 12	PROFESSOR JOHN OLIVER NELSON Yale "Are You Sure about That?"
November 19	PROFESSOR ROBERT L. CALHOUN Yale A United Ministry Forum

Minister—
Jackson Burns, 38 Langdon St., Cambridge — KI 7-5350

Minister to Students—
Paul Stopenhagen, 30 Langdon St., Cambridge — UN 4-1154

Minister's Assistant—
Mrs. R. G. Ramsdell, 9 Oxford St., Cambridge — EL 4-9019

Organist—
Richard G. Appel, 15 Hilliard St., Cambridge — KI 7-9654

Choir Director—
Mrs. Alfred N. Patterson, 25 Brimmer St., Boston — RI 2-1676

Sexton—
Rudolph Kelsey, 18 Eliot St., Cambridge — EL 4-2630

Chapter 5.

"What we need now is a great man…"

OPINIONS AND ADVICE, 1952 WILL EXPRESSES VALUES

FROM CHAPTER II, ABOUT Uncle Charlie's personality traits seen in his handwriting (rightward slanted strokes), he was prone to express his feelings; and, his reported behavior leaves little doubt. Sister Nancy recalled on her 1952 trolley trip with Uncle Charlie, he reprimanded smoking passengers with a very public announcement—"No Smoking."

During the 1952 Korean War period, when asked by a reporter his views on politics, Uncle Charlie empathetically responded, "What we need now is a great man who shall say what needs to be done and will do it. Senator Taft (Ohio) makes a good senator but he's not the man we need for this terrible situation." It's now 2014, and history seems to be repeating itself. I say AMEN.

More on politics, 1952: "He hopes that General MacAuthur will be the candidate, but expects it will be Eisenhower. He chose General Grant for his first presidential election vote. 'He was a great general, but not a good administrator. Eisenhower and MacAuthur are exceptions to that rule.'"

Uncle Charlie further noted, "A good citizen ought to be interested

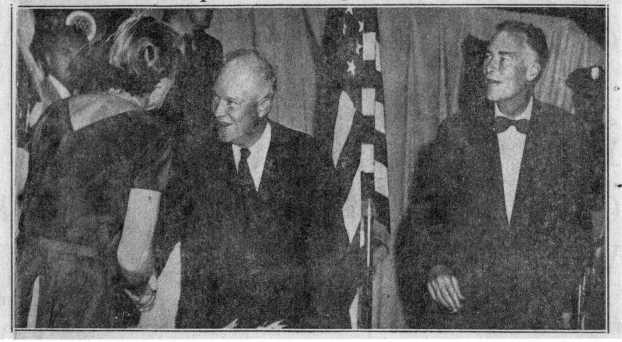

President Eisenhower and Governor Christian Herter attended the 1953 Massachusetts Republican Club banquet where Uncle Charlie was recognized as the oldest Republican among 5000 attendees.

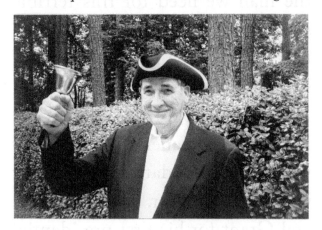

in politics, enough bad citizens already are."

Note: Josh ran for State of Georgia Insurance Commissioner, as a Libertarian candidate, in 1998. Josh is happy he lost.

Uncle Charlie on the military: "If I had my way, I'd have every young man and woman get into the military where they'd learn discipline… and how to concentrate their minds on their jobs."

On Marriage: "But, how would you know if she was the right one until after the wedding?"

On Alfred Kinsey, 1953: "He's just trying to get people all stirred up so they'll buy his book. He isn't saying anything new." Note: Kinsey

48

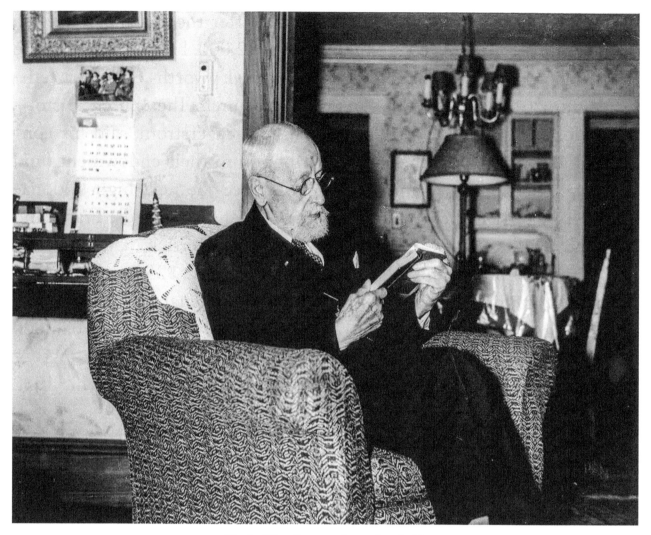

Uncle Charlie consulting his Bible.

authored books about human male and female sexuality.

Financial success: "I'm pleased I was a success in every business I tried." In Chapter VIII, Josh recounts his success record.

On smoking and drinking Uncle Charlie frequently said, "Don't smoke, don't drink, and do what the Bible says." Uncle Charlie taught an all boys Sunday school class at his Church. He spotted one of his charges smoking a cigarette in Harvard Square. He walked up to him, took the cigarette out of his mouth, and threw it in the gutter.

Uncle Charlie's 1952 Will & 1954 Codicil clearly expressed his values. It detailed, at length, specific bequests to many charitable causes. For example, the Cambridge Home for the Aged, $2,000 (this is about $18,000 inflation adjusted for 2013); the Mount Auburn Hospital, $3,000 ($27,000 in 2013 dollars); The Preacher's Aid Society, $2,000. The Cambridge YMCA, $2,000, to help liquidate its debt. Nieces Helen Giddings and Carrie Batchelder: the will stated, "I leave nothing." He apparently didn't agree with their values. To nephew, Raymond Thiery, to whom he had given $2,000 for a big legal problem he gave 1/7 of the residual estate (after the specific bequests), minus $2,000. He gave stock to the Harvard-Epworth United Methodist Church. The church Historian, Lisa Fagerstrom, said his contribution to their endowment fund was "twice the next highest donation." To his landlords, Frank and Elizabeth Merrick, Uncle Charlie bequeathed $25 per week. His 1954 codicil changed that bequest to a single lump sum of $25,000 ($220,000 in 2013 dollars).

Note: The first page of his 1952 will follows.

I, Charles W. Thiery of Belmont, Middlesex County, Massachusetts, being of sound mind and memory, declare this to be my last will and testament, hereby revoking all testamentary instruments heretofore made by me.

1. I nominate, constitute and appoint the Harvard Trust Company of Cambridge, said County, to be executor of this my last will and testament, and I give it as such executor all powers with reference to the management, investment, conversion and sale of my estate or any part thereof, whether consisting of real, personal or mixed property, which I should have if personally present and acting.

2. To my niece Mrs. Marie Tufts of Wellesley Hills, Norfolk County, Massachusetts, and my nephew Louis S. Thiery of said Cambridge, I give and bequeath all my clothing, furniture, pictures and all other personal effects of any and every description, excepting out thereof my books and the three cases containing part thereof, as more fully set out in Paragraph 3 of this my last will and testament, the property so given and bequeathed to be disposed of as the said Mrs. Marie Tufts and the said Louis S. Thiery may see fit, and without their being in any way accountable to my estate, to my executor or to any one else for such disposition.

3. To John MacKinnon of 120 Avon Hill Street, said Cambridge, I give and bequeath the three book-cases, all the books contained therein, and in addition, such other of my books as may be found in my room at 121 Hammond Road, said Belmont.

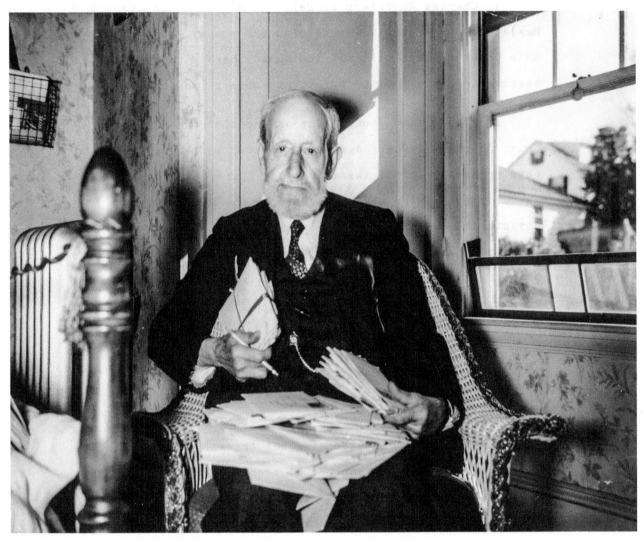

Uncle Charlie received hundreds of cards from well wishers

Chapter 6.
Playing the Age Card?
A Celebrated Centenarian (1850-1958)

"YOU DON'T HAVE TO do anything; you don't have to be famous. You go about your life, day by day, and then one day you reach 100, and everybody comes to see you!"

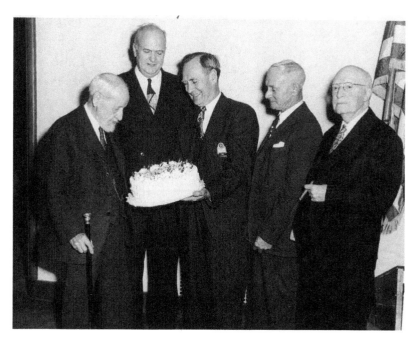

On reaching 100, the Rotary Club presented Uncle Charlie with a birthday cake.

Town Honors Charles Thiery, 100 Years O

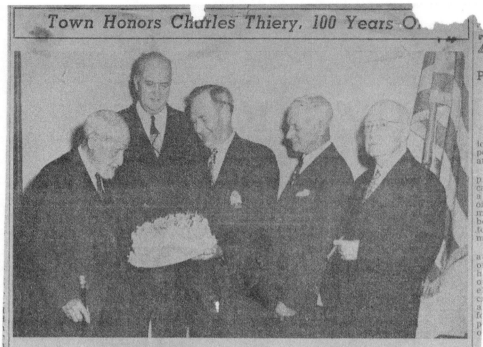

The Belmont Rotary Club and Town Officials honored Belmont's oldest resident, Charles Wesley Thiery, as he observed his 100th birthday yesterday. In excellent health, he's seen daily about town and on trips which he frequently makes unaided to Boston.

Mr. Thiery is shown on the left receiving a birthday cake from the hands of E. Robert Higgs, president of Rotary. Also shown (left to right) are Selectmen Howard D. Sharpe and Charles R. Betts, and a friend of 65 years' standing, Walter F. Beetle, who is nearing his 94th birthday.

Charles Wesley Thiery of 121 Hammond road reached the ripe old age of 100 years yesterday amidst considerable festivity and well-wishes.

This grand old man, whose appearance and agility belie his age by forty years, retired from business at the age of 93 and has been making his home in Belmont with Mr. and Mrs. L.

ELECTRICAL CONTRACTOR

Wiring for Light, Heat, Power
Residential work a specialty

HENRY A. HUGHES
280 Cross St.   BElmont 5-2682

Your fall clothes will look like new
when TAILOR FINISHED by

Edward's Tailoring

(Formerly G. A. DeLeso
Expert Tailoring, Alterations,

Frank Merrick ever since.

A long list of activities have been carried out in his honor during the week, starting at the Harvard-Epworth Methodist Church on Sunday with a special service. On Tuesday, Rotarians presented him with a huge birthday cake and town officials gave him the cherished Boston Post gold-headed cane.

During the remainder of the week he has been the honored guest at several gatherings and functions given him by friends and neighbors and was the recipient of a bouquet of 100 roses from the Cambridge lodge of Odd Fellows, of which he has been an active member.

The letter carrier brought to his home over 200 cards and letters yesterday, and he received

100TH BIRTHDAY
(Continued on Page 3 Col. 4)

many floral tributes and telegrams. Neighbors arranged a birthday supper last night.

Wednesday night he was the guest of the Republican Club of Massachusetts.

Payson Hall was filled when the Rotary Club staged a special program in Mr. Thiery's honor. He was introduced by Gordon B. Seavey, who also introduced a friend of Mr. Thiery's for 65 years, 93-year-old Walter F. Beetle.

In responding to the gift of the cane and the gold-encrusted birthday cake, Mr. Thiery said that it was only four years ago that he realized that he was getting old, when he counted a bouquet of 96 roses, symbolic of a rose for each year of his life . . . a year of 365 days, of 24 hours each.

Presentation of the cane, which had been handed down by several other old Belmontians, including David Chenery, Andrew J. McGinnis, and William P. Sanderson, was made on behalf of the town by Selectman Charles R. Betts.

Charles Wesley Thiery was born on Tremont street, Cambridge, October 26, 1850, and was named after the famous hymn writer. His mother died while he was still a boy and from time to time he was out of school to help in his father's watchmaking shop.

His father's solemn warning that "whatsoever a man soweth that shall he also reap" had an important effect in shaping his life.

Mr. Thiery began his business career as a watch case maker and later took up gold refining. His advice to modern business-

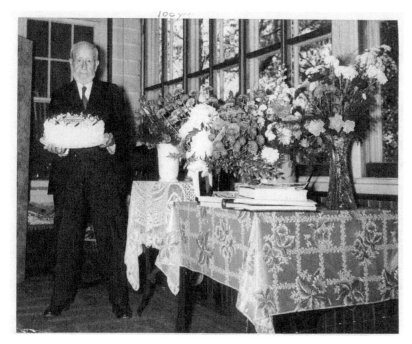

LEFT: Uncle Charlie at the Harvard Epworth United Methodist Church where a service was held in celebration of his 100th birthday.

Church to Honor Oldest Member

The Harvard-Epworth Methodist Church, Cambridge, will observe Charles Wesley Thiery Sunday, tomorrow to honor its oldest member on his 100th birthday. The Rev. Jackson Burns, pastor, will preach on the subject "I Am Not Ashamed of the Gospel," using the text chosen by Mr. Thiery.

Miss Marie Jean de Haller, traveling secretary for the World Student Christian Federation, who is paying a brief visit to this country, will be the speaker at 7:45 o'clock Sunday evening at the Wesley Foundation student meeting.

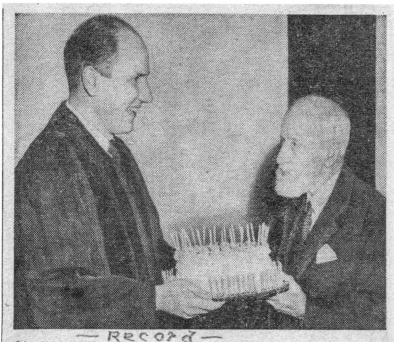

— Record —

Charles W. Thiery, Belmont, right, oldest member of the Harvard-Epworth Methodist Church, Cambridge, gets birthday cake from Rev. Mr. Jackson Burns, pastor. Thiery will be 100 years old Thursday. Cake is adorned with 100 candles.

100-YEAR-OLD MAN HONORED

— POST —

Charles Thiery Member of Church 84 Years

Honored for 84 years of membership in the Harvard - Epworth Church, Harvard sq., Cambridge, and for reaching his 100th birthday, Charles Wesley Thiery was praised by the minister at the morning service yesterday for his "notable Christian life." At a public reception afterwards, he was presented a cake bearing 100 candles.

Uncle Charlie was a member of his church a total of 92 years (age 15 until his death at 107).

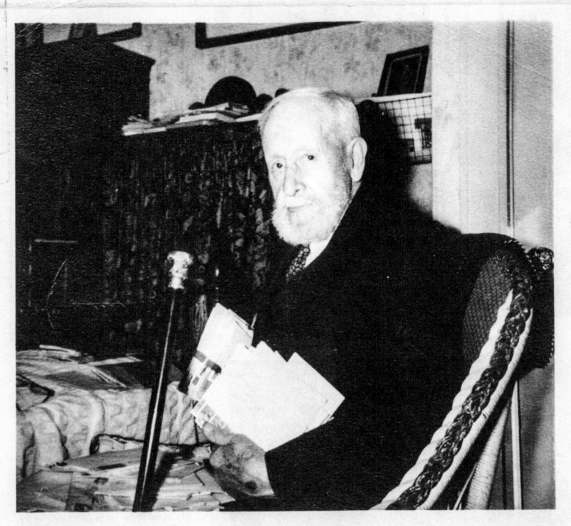

1850 - - - OCTOBER 26 - - - 1950

𝔚𝔦𝔰𝔥𝔦𝔫𝔤 𝔜𝔬𝔲 𝔞 𝔙𝔢𝔯𝔶 𝔐𝔢𝔯𝔯𝔶 𝔆𝔥𝔯𝔦𝔰𝔱𝔪𝔞𝔰

𝔞𝔫𝔡 𝔞

𝔥𝔞𝔭𝔭𝔶 𝔑𝔢𝔴 𝔜𝔢𝔞𝔯

CHARLES W. THIERY

Uncle Charlie's Christmas card sent when he was 100 years of age.

100-Year-Old Man Will Be Honored By Church Sunday

Suggests Text as Subject of Minister's Morning Sermon

Charles Wesley Thiery, who on October 26th will 100 years old, is to be honored at a special service a reception following the service at Harvard-Epwor Methodist church next Sunday morning at 11 a.m.

The Reverend Jackson Burns, pastor of the church, will preach on a text suggested by Mr. Thiery. His subject will be: "I Am Not Ashamed of the Gospel." Following the service, a reception will be held at which friends will have an opportunity to congratulate the oldest member of Harvard-Epworth church.

Mr. Thiery was born on Tremont st., Cambridge, near Hampshire st., on October 26, 1850. He attended the Webster school. He joined the Harvard Street Methodist church in 1866 and has been a member of that church, now united with Epworth church, since that time except for one brief period of a year and a half when he transferred his membership to a church in San Francisco. For 30 years he was a teacher in the Sunday school at Harvard Street church.

He began his career as a watch case maker and later took up gold refining. His advice to modern business men is "Always follow the Christian principles, On that principle and no other did I do business all my life."

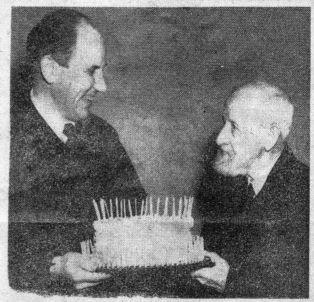

CAKE WITH 100 CANDLES is presented to Charles Wesley Thiery of Belmont, yesterday, by Rev. Jackson Burns of the Harvard-Epworth Methodist Church in Cambridge, where Mr. Thiery is oldest member. He will be 100 next Thursday.

Both the Boston Herald and Globe Newspapers covered Uncle Charlie

57

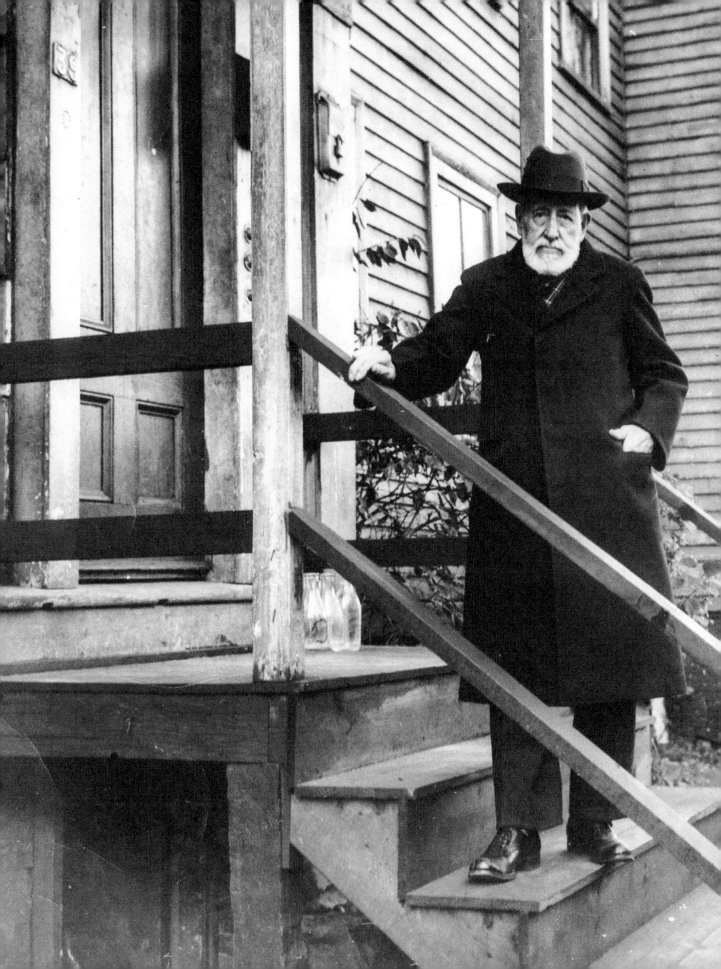

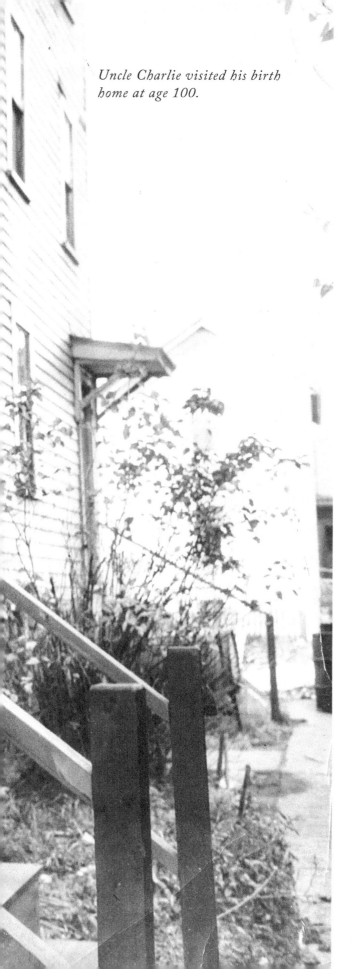

Uncle Charlie visited his birth home at age 100.

One Century Old

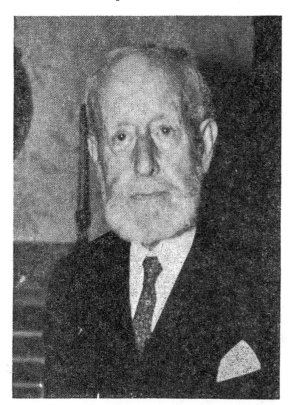

Tomorrow, October 26th, Mr. Charles Wesley Thiery of Belmont, Mass., will celebrate his 100th birthday. A member of the old Harvard Street Methodist Church, in Cambridge, since 1866, Mr. Thiery still retains a thoroughly active part in the work of Harvard-Epworth Church. He taught a Sunday School class there for 30 years. He attends services regularly, reads Zions Herald regularly, and expresses his opinions regularly. Last Sunday his fellow-Methodists in Cambridge honored him at a reception following the morning service. Mr. Thiery had chosen the text for the sermon and the Rev. Jackson Burns preached a challenging sermon on "I Am Not Ashamed of The Gospel."

Zions Herald and Methodism in general join in expressing very best wishes and congratulations to this sturdy servant of God whose life of devotion to the kingdom of God is a challenge to all men everywhere.

Five

Cambridge Church Honors Member 100 Years Old

Charles Wesley Thiery of 121 Hammond road, Belmont, who will be 100 years old Thursday, was honored at the morning service yesterday at the Harvard-Epworth Methodist Church, Cambridge, where he is the oldest member.

Thiery was born in Cambridge and was a Sunday School teacher

30 years. He joined the congregation 83 years ago. He is a retired watchmaker. His church endeavors were recounted by the minister, Rev. Jackson Burns. A reception followed the service.

E. German Official Flees Sector

BERLIN, Oct. 22 (Reuters)—Hermann Philipp, chief of the Forestry Department of the East German Agriculture Ministry has fled into the West Berlin sector, the West Berlin paper Tag said today.

Post Cane Awarded to Belmont Man, 100

GETS POST CANE IN BELMONT

Charles W. Thiery (centre) who will be 100 years old tomorrow, was presented the Boston Post cane last night at a pre-birthday reception tendered him at Payson Hall, Belmont. He's shown with Charles R. Betts (left) Belmont Selectman, and E. Robert Higgs, president of the Belmont Rotary Club.

Charles W. Thiery of 121 Hammond rd., Belmont, was awarded a Boston Post cane last night at a supper held in his honor by the Belmont Rotary Club at Payson Hall, Cushing sq., Belmont. Mr. Thiery will reach his 100th birthday tomorrow.

The cane was presented to him by Selectman Charles R. Betts of Belmont. A large cake was also prepared for the occasion by the members of the Rotary Club.

Mr. Thiery, who is a retired metalsmith, thanked the gathering of more than 100 businessmen and stated it was four years ago when he began to realize he was an old man. He attributes his long span of years to the fact that he has always remained single, with no wife to nag him.

amine the commission's records for payroll padding.

Their counsel, John A. Daly, filed a claim of exceptions in their behalf with the clerk of the court who informed him that his clients would have until Nov. 6 to complete and file their exceptions to the decision.

In granting Stevens' petition for a writ of mandamus, Judge Raymond S. Wilkins ruled that Stevens had a right, as a member of the commission, to examine the records in order to perform his duties properly. The court also ruled that Stevens should not have to wait until after election to make examination, but the notice of appeal given the court yesterday by the other members of the commission would indicate that Stevens will not be able to see the records

Will Observe 100th Birthday

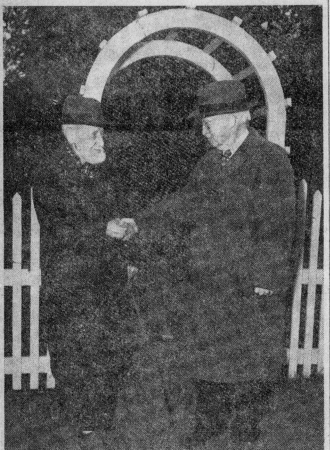

Belmont's "Grand Old Man," Charles W. Thiery (left) of 121 Hammond road, observes his 100th birthday next Thursday, October 26, with several parties during the week in his honor.

Extending him congratulations on approaching the century mark is a long-time friend, Walter F. Beetle of 21 Cushing avenue, who himself will observe his 94th birthday next spring. Both "old timers" are enjoying the best of health and are seen daily, rain or shine, around town.

Mr. Thiery, a bachelor, was born in Cambridge and lived there most of his life until coming to Belmont seven years ago to make his home with friends. He was a refiner of precious metals until his retirement at the age of 93.

All Belmont wishes him continued health and happiness for many more years to come.

(Hird photo)

Centenarian Says Hard Work Is No Killer

By ALTA MALONEY

"The strong die before the weak," says Charles W. Thiery of Belmont.

Thiery doesn't look like a weak man. His hand can give a crushing clasp, his body is erect and sturdy, his eyes are clear and his chin is firm and strong.

But Thiery says he never has been very well. And he thinks that this is why, on October 26, he will celebrate his 100th birthday.

ROSES DID IT

This rugged old Yankee, who comes from French, English and Dutch stock, found the idea of a newspaper interview amusing.

"You don't have to be famous, don't ever have to do anything," he said, smiling, "but you just keep going on from day to day, keep growing old. Then one day you're 100, and everybody comes to see you."

Four years ago, when he was 96, Thiery was honored by the Odd Fellows lodge. They called him

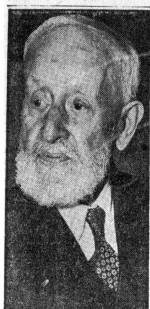

find few men who work as hard as I do."

Thiery likes alluding to Napoleon, who is one of his heroes. He keeps a shelf of books about the French emperor in his room and has a picture of him hung next to his bed, along with blown-up dauguerreotypes of his brother and himself as young men.

His brother died at 91, and one of his sisters, the strongest member of the family, died at 85.

FRETTED TOO MUCH

"She should have been alive today," Thiery says, "but she was always fretting and fuming. Thunder storms particularly would bother her. She wouldn't even let me open a window to get a little air.

"I'd say, 'Oh, a thunder storm —ain't that fine,' but she'd fuss. When she died, it was in the middle of a thunder storm."

The white-bearded, handsome old man relates instances when he was almost carried off. He doesn't remember the first occasion when he was being slowly starved. He was three days old and not getting enough nourishment from his milk. Three seed cakes from the corner store brought him out of that.

At two and a half he had pneumonia, but they didn't give him time to die. This, he believes, shrank his "bellows" so that several times he almost drowned for lack of wind.

Excessive swimming in the Charles near his boyhood home also gave him a mild attack of St. Vitus dance, a year he remembers with horror.

CENTURY MARK NEARS for Charles W. Thiery, retired businessman, of Belmont, who owes his long life, he feels, to never having felt very well.

up on the platform and presented a bouquet of 96 roses.

"I didn't make very much over it," he says. "I thanked them for it and went back to my seat.

"It wasn't until those roses opened out, full bloom, at home, and I looked at them and thought —each one of these stands for 365 days of 24 hours each—that I realized for the first time I was an old man."

Since he retired from his business, Thiery has lived with friends at 121 Hammond street, Belmont. Before that he always had lived in Cambridge, where he was born on Tremont street in a house which still stands.

He retired at 93, not because he was too old to work, but because his business—trading in gold—had petered out after the 1934 "gold rush" and supplies were coming in only by driblets.

This move was made against the advice of his doctor, who told him that if he gave up his business, he would die within a year. Thiery had noticed that in other people, so he has devoted himself to keeping busy, reading his books, which are stacked up everwhere in his room, taking walks, doing temperance and church work, taking a "decent citizen's interest" in politics.

COULDN'T KILL HIM

Another theory Thiery knocks down is that working under tension kills men young.

"I've been a driver for years and years," he dcelares emphatically. "I've reminded myself of Napoleon's army—always making a forced march. I'd start out on Monday morning under a strain and keep going under a strain. Sometimes it was 1:30 Sunday morning before I'd quit.

"Work don't kill a man. You'll

ALWAYS SUCCESSFUL

And when he left his outdoor life and started to work for his father in his watchcase making business, Thiery began having the digestive troubles which have plagued him ever since.

Looking back, Thiery is pleased that he has been a success in every business he has tried — watchcase manufacturing, which was ruined by the wrist watch; book selling, retail jewelry selling and finally as a gold dealer.

He left that last business because he was cheated so many times, but when he entered it again after requests from many customers, he realized that he had gone through all the frauds and had become an expert.

He began to be a financial success and, when he had more money than he needed for current expenses, he invested it safely. When he had enough, he retired.

The centenarian has another proud memory, that of being a corporal at 17 in the state cavalry, and he says: "If I had my way, I would have every young man and and woman get into the military, where they would learn discipline, be taught to obey orders and concentrate their minds on their jobs.

Mischievous himself up to 16, Thiery joined the Harvard Street Methodist Church and since then has not uttered but one oath, has never taken an alcoholic drink and has not smoked.

MISSED DANCING

He didn't know how to dance either, but he declares, "I was full of it as a boy and, if I had had a chance, I bet I would have." He never married.

Smoothing his soft white whiskers under his chin, he like to tell about the time he was fooling with other members of the cavalry and pretended that he was going to smoke a cigar.

A "sot" whom he had seen the night before, lying drunk with his feet out of his tent, caught hold of him and pleaded, "Don't, Charles, don't break your record."

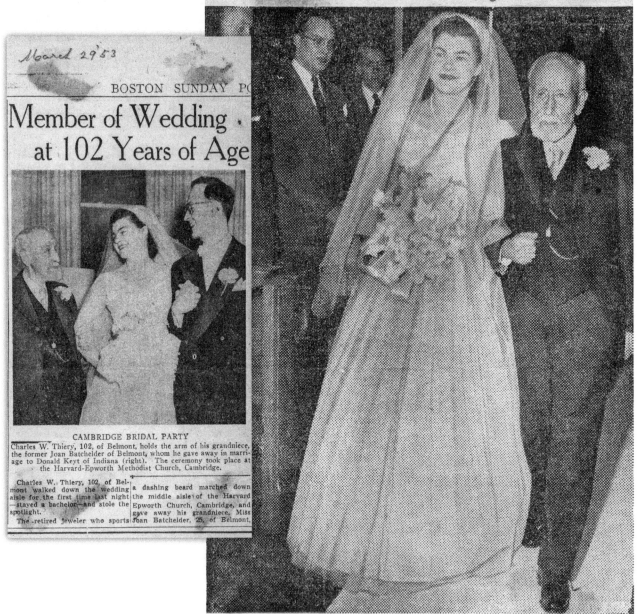

Gives Bride Away at 102

March 29 '53

BOSTON SUNDAY PO[ST]

Member of Wedding at 102 Years of Age

CAMBRIDGE BRIDAL PARTY

Charles W. Thiery, 102, of Belmont, holds the arm of his grandniece, the former Joan Batchelder of Belmont, whom he gave away in marriage to Donald Keyt of Indiana (right). The ceremony took place at the Harvard-Epworth Methodist Church, Cambridge.

Charles W. Thiery, 102, of Belmont walked down the wedding aisle for the first time last night —stayed a bachelor—and stole the spotlight.

The retired jeweler who sports a dashing beard marched down the middle aisle of the Harvard Epworth Church, Cambridge, and gave away his grandniece, Miss Joan Batchelder, 25, of Belmont,

DOWN THE AISLE of the Harvard-Epworth Church, Cambridge, go Joan Thierry Batchelder, of Belmont and Sudbury, and her 102-year-old grand-uncle, Charles Wesley Thierry of Belmont. "Uncle Charlie" gave the bride away at her marriage to Donald E. Keyt of Indianapolis.

Sunday Advertiser Photo by Bill Jones

Bachelor, 102, To Escort Bride

(Continued from First Page)

And he was. Two years after the war—the Civil War—Mr. Thiery joined the 1st Brigade, Boston Light Dragoons, served with them eight years and was mustered out a sergeant.

Miss Batchelder is quite thrilled to be given away by "Uncle Charlie," who is only 77 years older than she is. A junior at Boston University, she will become the bride of Donald E. Keyt, 25, son of Mr. and Mrs. Herbert C. Keyt of 2224 Langley Rd., Indianapolis, Ind.

The prospective bridegroom is an Arthur Little Co. engineer and is studying for his master's degree at M.I.T. Miss Batchelder explained that her twin brothers, Joshua Henry and Donald Richard, are at Air Force bases in Texas and her third brother, John MacCauley, is a Marine captain in Puerto Rico.

Mr. Thiery is as thrilled as Joan is. "I'm proud of that girl," he said.

The ceremony will be at 7:30 p.m. in the Harvard-Epworth Church in Harvard Square where Mr. Thiery has attended for 86 years. He'll be in a cutaway — "I gues you call them a Prince Albert. Last time I wore it was at a wedding."

Wedding guests really should have something to see. Not only a bright bride but at her side Mr. Thiery, five-feet, two inches tall, white-bearded and looking as though he just stepped out of a Victorian bandbox.

NOT "SOCIETY MAN"

Asked: "Are you fond of weddings?" Mr. Thiery told The Herald: "Not particularly. I'm not a society man, you know. I'm a plain home man."

For a plain home man Mr. Thiery has been the wonder of the neighborhood for years now. Many times he's been seen chasing a street car and catching it.

He once said his long life was due to hard work and "having a very bad stomach." Seems that made him watch his diet and take more care of himself than most of us.

He didn't retire until he was 93 after many years in such businesses as making watch cases and trading in gold.

A modest man, Mr. Thiery will twinkle when he tells you he lays claim to only three virtues— "never smoked, never drank and always voted Republican, except for Blaine in 1884."

Step out in
NEW YORK'S
EASTER PARADE

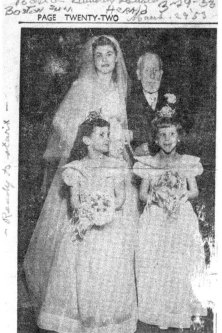

Boston Sunday Herald 3-29-53
Boston Herald March 29 '53

PAGE TWENTY-TWO

~ Ready to retire ~

GIVING AWAY his grandniece yesterday at Harvard-Epworth Church, Harvard square, was Charles Wesley Thiery, 102, of Belmont, who is standing beside the bride, Joan Batchelder of 123 Hammond St. In front, left to right, are the flower girls, Johanna E. Cross, 5, and Sharon Lee Taylor, 7. The bridegroom was Donald E. Keyt of Indianapolis, Ind.

(Herald Staff Photo by Russ Adams)

BACHELOR, 102, AT ALTAR --TO GIVE BRIDE AWAY

Charles Wesley Thiery, 102, late a sergeant of the Light Dragoons and as cavalier a bachelor as ever braved a wedding march last night walked up to the altar for the first time in all those 102 years.

Bachelor "Uncle Charlie" gave away the bride, his grandniece, Miss Joan Thiery Batchelder, 25, of 123 Hammond St., Belmont, in her marriage to Donald E. Keyt, 25, M.I.T. graduate student.

Miss Batchelder was a most fair bride and all eyes of the more than 200 guests in the Harvard-Epworth Church were on her most of the time, of course.

But for the rest of the time the eyes were on "Uncle Charlie" because, after all, there's something about an old soldier.

"Uncle Charlie" wore a cutaway and in his buttonhole was a bright carnation and when he walked the aisle he did it with all the spring of a bridegroom.

Asked: "How does it happen that you never married?" "Uncle Charlie" said: "I had to stick to business. Father's business was in a precarious state when I went into it."

All the guests agreed that if the rest of the brigade were like "Uncle Charlie" then it would have been something to see a charge of the Light Dragoons.

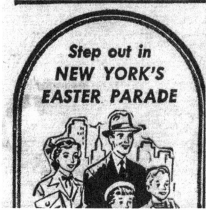

Wedding Duty for Light Dragoon

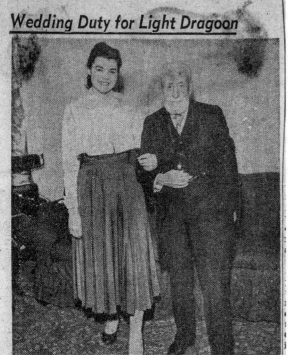

(Herald Staff Photo by Ernest MacLean)

THE BACHELOR AND THE BRIDE—At 102 years of age Charles Wesley Thiery trips down the aisle next Saturday to give in marriage his grandniece, Miss Joan Thiery Batchelder. Says he won't be nervous because he's an old military man.

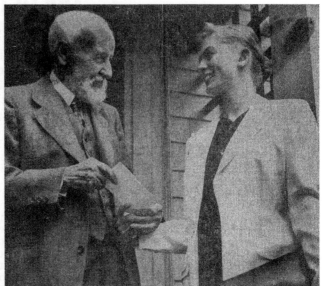

EISENHOWER DINNER HELPERS get together in Belmont as Patty Flett, 18, gives Charles W. Thiery, 102, an invitation to the dinner which will be held at Boston Garden, Sept. 21.

Uncle Charlie, 102, Will Escort Bride

By FRED BRADY

On this Saturday night Charles Wesley Thiery, 102 years old, gives a last pat to his trim beard, sticks a fresh posy in his buttonhole and then—with all the military dash of a Light Dragoon—walks a wedding march with a pretty girl on his arm.

★ ★ ★

No, he is not sacrificing 102 years as a bachelor. But he is giving the bride away.

She is his grandniece, Miss Joan Batchelder of 123 Hammond St., Belmont, whose mother is widowed and whose three brothers are away in the service and couldn't get home to do the honors.

★ ★ ★

Mr. Thiery is happy to do them. The Herald asked: "Think you'll be nervous?" Mr. Thiery came right back with: "I don't see any reason why I should. I used to be a military man."

64

Youth And Age Enthusiastic For Ike Dinner

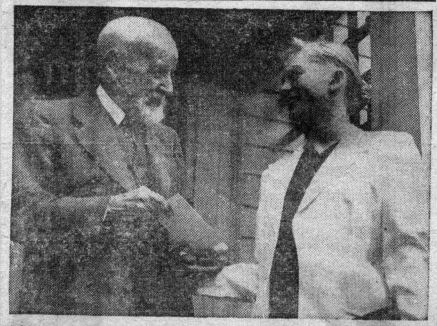

Eighteen-year-old Patty Flett of Belmont presents an invitation to the Eisenhower Dinner to her 102-year-old neighbor, Charles W. Thiery. Though there is an 84 year difference in their ages, both are enthusiastic workers for the dinner which will be held at the Boston Garden, Monday evening, September 21st. Committees from all six New England States will co-operate on this first all-New England dinner reception ever given to a President of the United States.

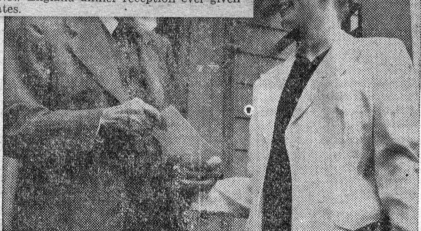

YOUNG AND OLD — ENTHUSIASM SHOWN FOR IKE DINNER. Eighteen-year-old Miss Patty Flett, daughter of Selectman and Mrs. J. Watson Flett of 184 Rutledge road, presents an invitation to the Eisenhower dinner to Charles W. Thiery, age 102, of 121 Hammond road, who has voted "Republican" ever since he cast his first vote for General Grant in 1872.

Though there is an eighty-four year difference in their ages, both are enthusiastic workers for the dinner which will be held at the Boston Garden, Monday evening, September 21. Committees from all six New England States will cooperate on this first all-New England Dinner reception ever given to a President of the United States.

Don't Marry; Follow Bible

Belmont Man, 103, Ready to Tell Ike His Formula at Hub Dinner

A Belmont man who was born when 13th President Millard Fillmore was in the White House is going to shake hands next Monday with 34th President Dwight Eisenhower.

And if Mr. Eisenhower wants

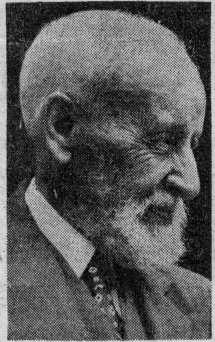

"I NEVER MET A PRESIDENT," says Charles W. Thiery, 103, of Belmont.

to know how to live to be 100, Charles W. Thiery will be ready to tell him. Thiery already has turned the trick and is working

on his second century. He'll be 103 next month, he told the United Press. What is Thiery's formula for long life? Briefly this:

Don't get married; don't use liquor; don't use tobacco; do what the Bible says.

Whenever he's in doubt, the centenarian consults his Bible.

"A good many more people nowadays would live to be my age if they followed the Book. Go to God. You'll get the right answer."

Clear of eye, his thatch of white hair thinning on top and wearing a full white beard, Thiery looks more like a well-preserved man of 80 than a centenarian. He thinks nothing of walking half a mile to a car stop two or three times a week to go to Boston.

Thiery, who didn't retire as a gold buyer until he was 92, had these observations:

On politics—"A good citizen ought to be interested in politics. Enough bad citizens are already."

On Kinsey—"He's just trying to get people all stirred up so they'll buy his book. He isn't telling anything new."

Right now, Thiery is looking forward to attending a $100-a-plate Republican dinner in Boston Monday and shaking hands with President Eisenhower.

"I've never met a President," he said. "But I got a good look at General Grant when I was in the militia back in 1866."

In Harmony

All in harmony, President Eisenhower, Governor Herter and Senator Saltonstall, l. to r., present studies in serious mien as Saltonstall spoke during the Chief Executive's appearance in Boston yesterday. Radio and TV carried the President's message throughout the nation.

(Record-American Photo, John Murphy)

➤——————————→

Admiration

Charles W. Thiery, 103, great admirer of President Eisenhower, shown with his grandniece, Nancy Batchelder of South Sudbury, Mass., was among those attending Ike's Boston Garden reception last night. Thiery, a resident of Belmont, voted for Ike in the last election, just as he voted for every Republican since Pres. Grant except Blaine.

(Story on Page 2)

(Record-American Photo, John Murphy)

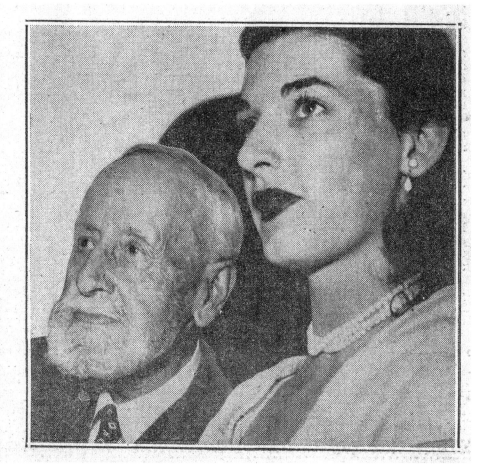

103-Year-Old Introduced

And like the rest, the President smiled and shook his head in amazement when Gov. Herter, the toastmaster, introduced 103-year-old Charles Thiery of Belmont, who stood proudly and acknowledged the plaudits of the crowd.

With the 5000 others, the President bowed his head for 15 seconds in a tribute to Senator Taft. It was said that the homage to Taft was the suggestion of President Eisenhower.

During the "speech-making," which preceded his own, the President was attentive to each of the Republican leaders. He applauded each generously, as did the throng.

As the clock moved relentlessly towards the moment he was to

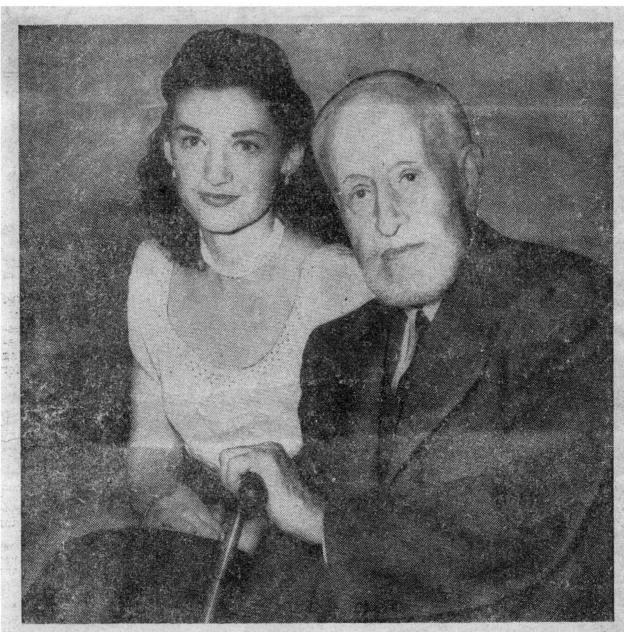

OLDEST REPUBLICAN AT BANQUET—Charles W. Thiery, 103, of Belmont, who first voted for President Grant, attends dinner to Ike with grandniece, Nancy Batchelder of South Sudbury.

ADDRESS OF THE PRESIDENT
   AT THE BOSTON GARDEN, BOSTON MASS.

   SEPTEMBER 21, 1953
   9:30 p.m., e.d.s.t.

AS ACTUALLY DELIVERED
_____

MY FELLOW AMERICANS:

        After the embarrassing generosity of the compliments that have
been paid me this evening from this platform, you can well understand
that I am in some danger of thinking a little too well of myself. Thank
goodness, many years ago, I had a preceptor, for whom my admiration has
never died, and he had a favorite saying, one that I trust I try to live
by. It was: always take your job seriously, never yourself.

        Now, in spite of this embarrassment, I would like on this occasion
and in front of this audience, to say just a word of my obligation to some
of the political leaders that have appeared here this evening, and who do
us so much honor by their presence.

        I have just been introduced by Senator Saltonstall, the Chairman
of the great National Defense Senate Committee, and as such a crucial and
key figure in that great body. Very naturally, I am happy to be with my
colleague and old friend, Chris Herter, your Governor, whom I expect again
to be Governor. And then John Lodge, Governor of Connecticut, and
Governor Cross of Maine -- and I shall not forget it is the Northeastern
of our States. And Senator George Aiken, Chairman of that great
Agricultural Committee; and Secretary of Commerce, my colleague in
Washington, Sinclair Weeks. And of course, every day each of us has many
reasons for feeling indebted to Ambassador Henry Cabot Lodge for his work
in the United Nations.

        Of course, I cannot possibly list all of the great individuals
who are here this evening, but certainly I must mention my friend Governor
Gregg of New Hampshire, and Lieutenant Governor Johnson, Senator Flanders;
and finally I think there must be something unique that we can have here
on the platform this evening both the present and the future Speaker of
the House of Representatives in Washington, and the present and the next
President Pro Tem of the Senate.

        I suggest that a list of names such as I have just recited gives
some idea of the brilliance of the political leadership that this great
section of our country -- the thumb of our country, if your please -- has
produced. I pay here my tribute to them.

        Now, ladies and gentlemen, the Republican Party is nearing the
100th Anniversary of its founding.

        Now, we would be wise, I think, to recall briefly the
circumstances of that event, just a few months short of 100 years ago.
It came with the meeting of a small group of rebellious Whigs and
disenchanted Democrats in the little town of Ripon, Wisconsin. Other
towns, understandably coveting the honors of history, dispute the
particular claim of this Wisconsin community. And indeed political
dissent and disillusion were seething in those years far across town
limits and state borders. Everywhere the tremors of a divided nation
were felt. To many, the drift toward civil war seemed fatefully sure.
But there is no dispute as to the purpose inspiring the many groups who
reached for a new hope and a new party which they called Republican.
That purpose, everywhere plainly defined and passionately proclaimed,
was to halt the extension of the institution of slavery.

69

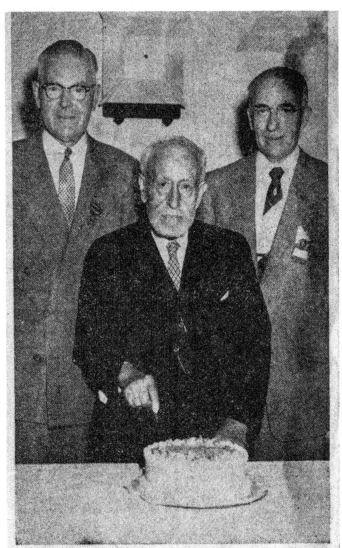

HONORARY ROTARIAN AT 105 YEARS of age is Charles Wesley Thiery, who was given this honor on the occasion of his 105th birthday by Belmont Rotarians. Shown with Mr. Thiery cutting his birthday cake are Rotary President John A. Collins and Vice-President Earle M. Prescott.   (Hird photo)

Dr. White Relays Ike's Salute to Mr. Thiery, 105

Greetings from President Eisenhower were among the hundreds of congratulatory messages received by Charles W. Thiery as he observed his 105th birthday Wednesday.

From his hospital room at Denver, the President sent his best wishes to Belmont's agile centenarian-plus through Dr. Paul Dudley White, who relayed them when he paid an hour's personal visit to Mr. Thiery at his home, 121 Hammond rd., that evening.

Mr. Thiery, the oldest member of the Republican Club of Massachusetts, recently sent a birthday message and wishes for a speedy recovery to the President. In conversations with his distinguished patient, Dr. White also had told the Chief Executive of the remarkable Mr. Thiery, whom he has frequently introduced to groups of doctors and medical students as an outstanding example of how long a man can live with a mild heart condition.

Dr. White also presented to Mr.

(Continued on Page 2, Col. 8)
over

70

OFFICE OF THE VICE PRESIDENT
WASHINGTON

October 21, 1955

Dear Mr. Thierry:

It is with a great deal of pleasure that Mrs. Nixon and I join your relatives and friends from all parts of the world in extending our greetings and very best wishes to you as you celebrate your 105th birthday on October 26.

I understand that you are a staunch Republican and I want you to know that it gives all of us great courage to know that a person of your years and wisdom has been such a good supporter of our party throughout the years.

May you continue to be blessed with health, happiness and warm friendships.

Sincerely,

Richard Nixon

Mr. Charles W. Thierry
121 Hammond Road
Belmont, Massachusetts

Heart of a Boy, Says Dr. White
Belmont Youth, 106, Hailed

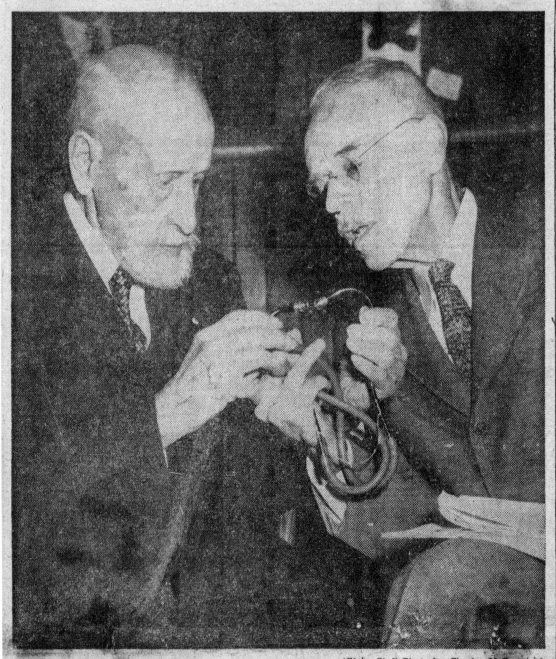

(Globe Staff Photo by Charles McCormick)

NOT TOO OLD TO WALK A MILE A DAY, "except when it's raining," Charles Theiry (left) told Dr. Paul Dudley White today. Mr. Theiry is 106 years old and lives at 106 Hammond rd., Belmont. Here he examines Dr. White's gold stethoscope.

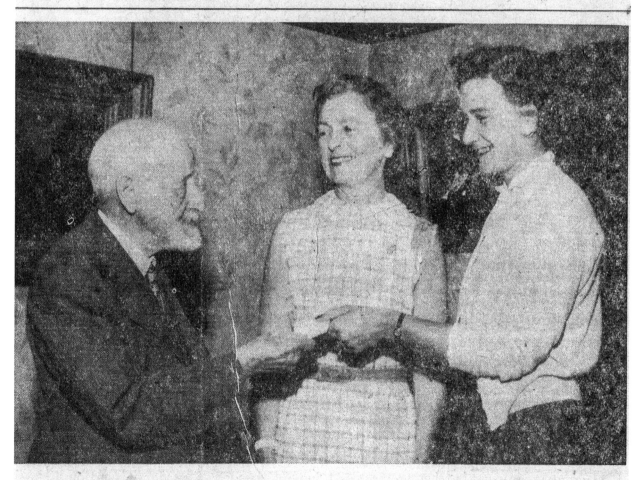

"WE'RE NEVER TOO OLD to help a cause we believe in," says Charles W. Thiery of Belmont, who will be 106 next month. Mr. Thiery is the oldest member of the Republican Club of Massachusetts. He cast his first vote for General Grant in 1872. He is shown here making a $100 contribution to the Massachusetts Republican Campaign Fund. Accepting on behalf of the party are, Mrs. Leland G. Darrow (center) of Harwich Port and Belmont, party finance chairman for the town of Belmont and Miss Priscilla H. Winters, of Belmont, representing the Republican State Committee.

loor
the
ond
mes
vic-
s he
rom
In-

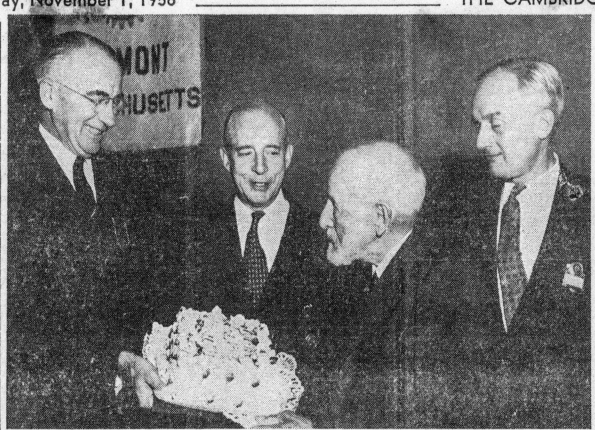

106 YEARS OLD: Charles Wesley Thiery, who was born at 39 Tremont st., this city, reached his 106th birthday on October 26. The Belmont Rotary Club, of which he is an honorary member, presented him with a colorful birthday cake. Dr. Earle M. Prescott, president, is shown making the presentation, as District Governor Fred H. Nickels and Vice President Ralph D. Stauffer look on. A bachelor and retired gold refiner, Mr. Thiery has been a member of Harvard-Epworth Methodist Church, Cambridge, for 89 years. He is in the best of health and still takes a brisk daily walk. The oldest member of the Republican Club of Massachusetts, he first voted for General Grant in 1872 and is anticipating casting his ballot in next Tuesday's Presidential election. (Photo courtesy of Belmont Citizen).

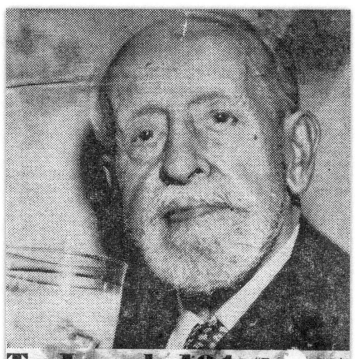

To Reach 104

"D... get marr... ...use liquor or tobacco. Do what the Bible says," and you may live to 104, like Charles W. Thiery, of Belmont, Mass. —AP

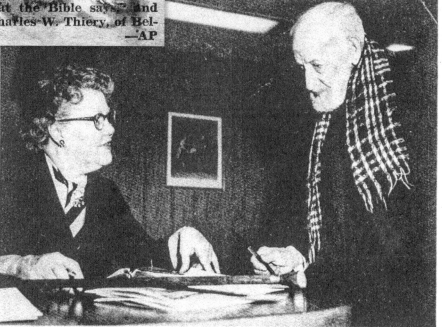

YANKEE CENTENARIAN — Charles W. Thireay of Belmont, shown registering with Observation Area Receptionist Mrs. Ida Wilson, is 106 years old — 11 years older than the John Hancock! Mr. Thireay visited the 26th Floor last week, and is believed to be the oldest man to ever tour the top of the Home Office. Mr. Thireay once served in the Boston Light Dragoons of the State Cavalry, and in professional life was a manufacturer of gold and silver watchcases. When asked to what he attributed his longevity, he summed up the situation in four words: "I . . . am a bachelor."

TO OBSERVE 107TH BIRTHDAY

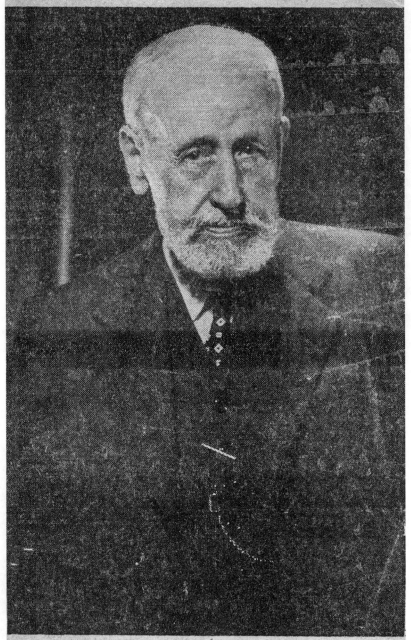

CHARLES W. THIERRY

(Photo by Martin Cornel)

107 YEARS YOUNG ... Belmont's oldest living resident, sprightly Charles W. Thierry of 121 Hammond Rd. will celebrate his 107th birthday on October 26. Still hale and hearty, Mr. Thiery can be seen most any good day walking around Cushing Square. A lifelong Republican and a bachelor, gives a lot of credit for his longevity to a sensitive stomach that made him very careful of his diet. He was honored yesterday by the Retired Men's Club of the Belmont Methodist Church and for the seventh consecutive year, Mr. Thierry will be the guest of honor next Tuesday night at the Belmont Rotary Club. A special birthday cake will be baked for the occasion.

The Best Advice Is to Stay Healthy

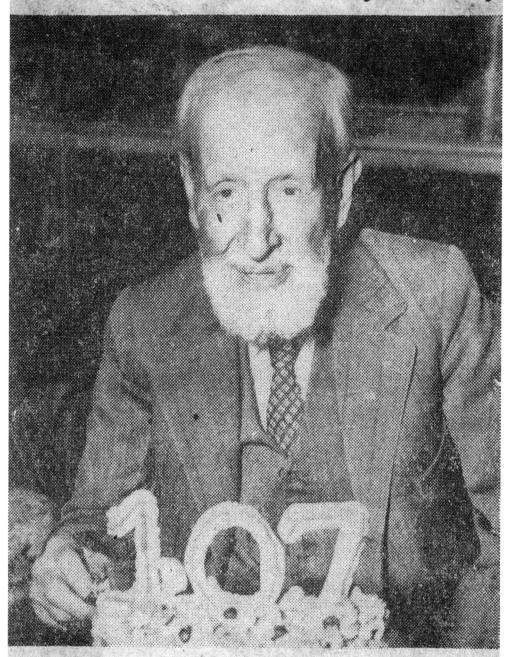

(Associated Press Wirephoto)

Belmont—Charles Wesley Thiery beams happily as he cuts a cake in honor of his 107th birthday. Outside of pneumonia when he was 2 years old, and a "slow fever" at 20, Thiery never has had anything wrong with him. He wears glasses to read and write and uses a cane on frequent solo trips to Boston. He offers no special advice for a long life except to stay healthy.

No Thiery Theory

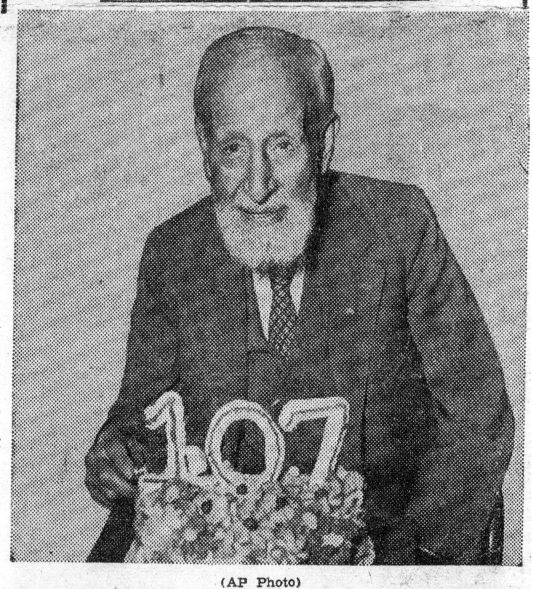

(AP Photo)

CHARLES WESLEY THIERY of Belmont celebrates his 107th birthday today. Thiery says he has no special recipe or theory for long life.

Uncle Charlie Old Timers

(See Photo Right Below)

The term Old Timer is relative. A ten year old looks on a high school boy as an old timer. The class of 1933 is tottering on the brink of senility, to the entering freshman. Meetings of the Boston Market Gardeners Association are apt to bring out old timers — Charley Wyman, for example. He in turn points to one who certainly is entitled to the classification and at a BMGA meeting showed us a photograph of himself with this friend who is 107 years old. Charles Wesley Thiery is the world's oldest Rotarian. He retired at 93 from his business of gold refining because there wasn't much old gold around. "I have had to watch what I eat," he says, "and always have had to take good care of myself." He is a bachelor; never smoked or drank; is a life-long Republican (remembers voting for General Grant). He has lived most of his life in Belmont, Mass.; makes his home with a couple in their Eighties. He calls them "the young folks."

Wymans of Arlington

Charley (Charles F.) Wyman too is "young folks" to Mr. Thiery. The Wyman family were pioneers and leaders in market gardening. Two brothers, Frank and Dan, started the Wyman farm which, with its greenhouses, was a well known landmark, on Lake street, Arlington, Mass. Frank Wyman was Charley's father. At the same market gardeners' meeting where we picked up the Thiery-Wyman photo, a pair of strong hands suddenly gripped our shoulders. We thought, "What youngster is that?" They were the hands of M. Ernest Moore who is over eighty — an Old Timer. But many a young man couldn't match that grip.

As we go to press (March 17) news comes of Mr. Thiery's death.

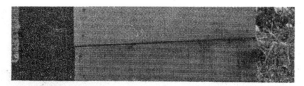

CONTINUING OUR SERIES OF UN-USUAL RFD BOXES — the postman says, "Well, well, well" when he comes to this trio in Lexington, Mass.

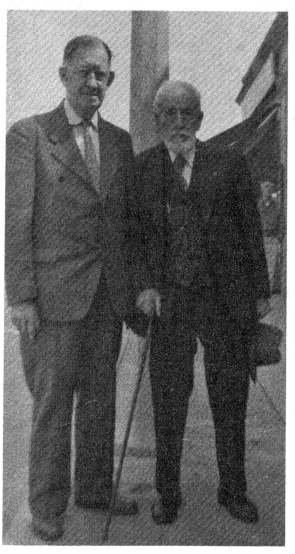

CHARLEY WYMAN WITH 107 YEAR OLD FRIEND.

es at 107 Years. —

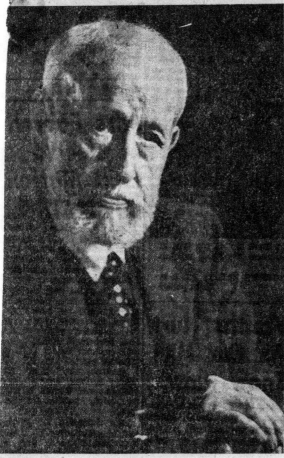

CHARLES WESLEY THIERY

(Continued from Page 1, Col. 6)

ucted Wednesday afternoon at he Harvard-Epworth Methodist Church in Cambridge by the Rev. W. Edge Dixon. Mr. Thiery as the oldest member of that church, the Harvard part of which he joined in 1866, ninety-two years ago. He served as a unday School teacher for bout thirty years.

Burial was in Cambridge emetery.

Mr. Thiery leaves a niece, rs. Nathaniel P. Tufts of ellesley Hills and three nep-ws, Charles E. Batchelder of Santa Ana, Calif., Louis S, Thierry of Cambridge and Dr. Raymond Thiery of West Bridgewater.

Descended from a line of French Huguenots, Mr. Thiery was born October 26, 1850, on Tremont st., Cambridge, and lived in that city and Belmont all his long life, except when he went to San Francisco in 1875 for about a year and a half.

Named after the famous Methodist hymn writer, Charles Wesley, he attended the Web-ster School in Cambridge, but from time to time was taken out of school to help in his fa-ther's watch shop. His mother died while he was still a boy and he himself barely survived pneumonia when he was two and one-half years old.

Never Married

He was a bachelor and never smoked or drank.

Mr. Thiery began his busi-ness career as a watch case

Timothy F. Toomey

Funeral services are to be held today at Gulfport, Fla., for Timothy F. Toomey, former-ly of 43 Vincent ave., who died at his home in that Florida city Tuesday, March 18.

Mr. Toomey, who lived in Belmont nearly 25 years, retired as a carrier in 1951 after 47 years service with the Post Of-fice Department.

He leaves his wife, Anna; a son, Edward of Cambridge; a daughter, Mrs. Helen Dunning of Rochester, Mich.; a sister, Mrs. Mary Mahoney of Allston, and a brother, John J. Toomey of Cambridge.

Start Adult Courses

Among recent registrants for courses at the Cambridge Cen-ter for Adult Education are Andrea Kazanjian, 27 Stone rd.; Dr. and Mrs. David J. Sen-cer, 14 Choate rd.; Robert B. Nix, 117 Alexander ave.; F. John O'Reilly, Jr., 63 Taylor rd. and Mr. and Mrs. John Hobbs, Jr., 56 Beatrice circle.

maker and later took up gold refining. He said he retired at 93 not because of age, but be-cause there wasn't much more old gold around.

In 1950, at 100, he was pre-sented with the Boston Post cane as the town's oldest resi-dent. He outlived the news-paper which originated the cane.

When he was 102, he escort-ed his grandniece, Joan Thiery Batchelder, to the altar when she became Mrs. Donald E. Keyt. The same year the Vet-eran Odd Fellows Association of Massachusetts made him their honorary chaplain.

In 1953, a month before his 104th birthday he received an ovation at a rally at the Boston Garden when Governor Herter introduced him as the oldest Republican present. Mr. Thiery cast his first ballot for U. S. Grant and defected from the party only when he failed to vote for Blaine for President. On his 100th birthday the Re-publican Club of Massachu-setts gave him a party as its oldest member.

Ike Sent Greetings

In 1955, from his hospital room in Denver, President Eisenhower sent 105th birthday greetings which were personally relayed to Mr. Thiery by Dr. Paul Dudley White, who was then in national prominence for his reports to the country on the President's progress in re-covery from his heart attack.

Mr. Thiery was taken to sev-eral medical meetings by Dr.

Rotary —

(Continued from Page 1, Col. 8)

After tracing the history of the Family Service Association of Greater Boston for the past 75 years, Mrs. Hunt pointed out how her work is an investment in the future. She cited sever-al cases, with names disguised, how Belmont Family Service helps people to work out their problems and troubles through the counseling by members in her organization.

The Belmont organization has been affiliated since 1954 with the Greater Boston asso-ciation, a Red Feather service.

A brief tribute was made in the memory of Charles W. Thiery, an honorary member of Belmont Rotary, who died on Sunday at the age of 107. On the occasion of his 100th birth-day on October 26, 1950, the club staged a big reception in his honor, and since then he has been especially recognized each following anniversary.

Walter H. Taft, executive vice-president of the Belmont Savings Bank and a former president of the Rotary Club in Belmont, will speak on the functions of a savings bank in a residential community at next week's meeting, to be held in Payson Hall.

White, who pointed out to doc-tors not only Mr. Thiery's age but his good health and reten-tion of all of his faculties when he was far past 100.

In 1956 the agile centenarian-plus was walking along the sidewalk on Washington st. Boston, when a jagged part of a glass jug fell from an upper story of a building and landed on his head. He was given two stitches at a hospital, sent home in a taxi, and the next day was back in Boston again.

Mr. Thiery's birthdays each year since he reached 100 came in for considerable community attention. He was a guest of the Belmont Rotary Club on several such occasions and last October the Retired Men's Club, of which he was an honorary member, also had a cake for him.

He became a master Mason in Amicable Lodge, A. F. & A. M. of Cambridge in 1878, and a Royal Arch Mason in Cam-bridge Royal Arch Chapter in 1880. He was believed to be the second oldest Mason in the world.

He also was a member of Friendship Lodge of Odd Fel-lows, in Cambridge for 70 years, lacking a few weeks, and was the oldest Odd Fellow in this state.

Chapter 7.

Oldest Mason, Methodist, Odd Fellow, Rotarian, and Republican

Uncle Charlie's Network— The 4th Centenarian Habit, Connections

CONNECTIONS WITH FAMILY, FRIENDS, your community, state, nation, and world, even pets, support survival and extend longevity. The U.S. Air Force Rule of 3 states you cannot survive a life threatening emergency event without the following in the given time spans:

- 3 seconds without spirit and hope
- 3 minutes without air
- 3 hours without shelter in extreme conditions
- 3 days without water
- 3 weeks without food
- 3 months without companionship or love

Thinking about Chapter XIII—How Long Will You Live? From Ben Sherwood's book, *The Survivors Club,* I took the survivor test for Uncle Charlie. Using handwriting analysis, quotes from interviews, and knowledge from newspaper articles and family lore I determined what his answers would be.

Uncle Charlie's principal survivor type is **The Believer.** Over and over his refrain was "go to God" which contributed to his long life. He went to his Bible for answers. His conversion to Christianity, at age 15, sustained him. The remaining four survivor types fit him as well. His determination, perseverance, aggressiveness, and domineering style qualify him as **The Fighter.** Recall he was known to have removed a cigarette from the mouth of one of his Sunday school students he spotted in Harvard Square and he then threw the butt into the gutter. Uncle Charlie can be considered to be **The Connector** because of his enduring church and social organization memberships. He also could be **The Thinker** because of his analytical problem solving style, along with his strong intuitive nature. He also possessed the traits that define **The Realist,** which include being factual, frank, exploratory, and systematic.

Of the twelve strengths that support his survivor profile, I chose adaptability to be the most important. Uncle Charlie needed to deal with the family's fading watch cover business due to fashion changing. Wrist watches became popular for women and then men as they were a necessity for WWI pilots. As a result, he switched to gold trading, which was subject to supply shortages. He became involved with bookselling and the jewelry business to generate income. He retired at age 93 due to the gold shortage at that time (1943). Uncle Charlie's other strengths included resilience, being fatalistic (accepting adversity), persistence, and determination. Faith, of course, was a central theme for him from age 15 on. Empathy for others is very evident in his handwriting's rightward slanted upstrokes; and, his charitable actions show he followed through helping family and worthy causes. Although Uncle Charlie's formal education was limited, his intelligence is evident by his voracious reading.

Uncle Charlie flowed (demonstrated fluidity) through his daily routine, pushed on with pride and persistence. He had an abundance of intuition which gave him an advantage in the business world and would be considered instinct in survival situations.

Uncle Charlie found love though his connections. Family, church, and club associations supplemented his life as a workaholic.

Uncle Charlie's ingenuity showed when he upped the price on his slow moving diamond rings. The price increase helped customers recognize that they were buying a higher quality product.

In addition to family, my connections over the years are military, community, and business related: The Air Force Association; Civil Air Patrol—Georgia Wing Aerospace Education; The Dekalb-Peachtree Senior Squadron; Certified Toastmaster; the Buckhead Optimist Club; the Roswell UMC Singles Group Programs Coordinator; Georgia Writers Association; Navy Flying Club; current involvement includes Northlake Tucker Kiwanis, Tucker Business Association (Senior Vice President); Civil Air Patrol; Dekalb Peachtree Senior Squadron; Silver Wings Fraternity; American Association of Handwriting Analysts (AAHA); American Handwriting Analysts Foundation (AHAF); Southeastern Handwriting Analysts (SEHA); The 59th Fighter Squadron Association; Air Force Navigator Observer Association (AFNOA); the Atlanta Chapter of the Financial Service Professionals (SFP). I cannot leave out our miniature black schnauzer, Kelly; she provides love and laughter.

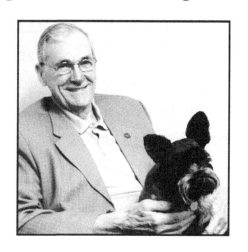

CLASS OF SERVICE

This is a full-rate Telegram or Cablegram unless its deferred character is indicated by a suitable symbol above or preceding the address.

WESTERN UNION (19)

W. P. MARSHALL, PRESIDENT

FX-1201

SYMBOLS

DL=Day Letter
NL=Night Letter
LT=Int'l Letter Telegram
VLT=Int'l Victory Ltr.

The filing time shown BB344 on telegrams and day letters is STANDARD TIME at point of origin. Time of receipt is STANDARD TIME at point of destination

B.CDU029 32 PD INTL=ZP FRANKFURTMAIN VIA WUCABLES 25=

:LT CHARLES W THIERY:

=121 HAMMOND RD BELMONT (MASS):

=GERMAN MASONS SEND GREETINGS AND CONGRATULATION TO THE

104 BIRTHDAY OF THE OLDEST FREEMASON OF THE WORLD=

:UNITED GRAND LODGE GERMANY DR THEODOR VOGEL

GRANDMASTER=

121 104=

THE COMPANY WILL APPRECIATE SUGGESTIONS FROM ITS PATRONS CONCERNING ITS SERVICE

In addition to family relationships, social and business affiliations help us to have a sense of importance and a reason to live. Another big benefit of being a member of a diverse number of groups is how much knowledge we can acquire from their teachings and from other individuals we meet within the membership.

WESTERN UNION

CLASS OF SERVICE

This is a full-rate Telegram or Cablegram unless its deferred character is indicated by a suitable symbol above or preceding the address.

1201

W. P. MARSHALL, PRESIDENT

SYMBOLS

DL=Day Letter

NL=Night Letter

LC=Deferred Cable

NLT=Cable Night Letter

Ship Radiogram

The filing time shown in the date line on telegrams and day letters is STANDARD TIME at point of origin.   Time of receipt is STANDARD TIME at point of destination

.•BA423

1950 OCT 21

B.NWA193 NL PD=NEWTON MASS 21=

CHARLES WESLEY THIERY (BETWEEN 10 AND 1030 AM)=

    CARE REV JACKSON BURNS HARVARD ETWORTH METHODIST

    CHURCH 1555 MASS AVE CAMBRIDGE MASS=

¶ "A GOOD NAME IS RATHER TO BE CHOSEN THAN GREAT RICHES AND

LOVING FAVOR RATHER THAN SILVER AND GOLD". YOU HAVE CHOSEN THE

BETTER PART. ON THIS AUSPICIOUS ANNIVERSARY, THE CENTENNIAL

OF A WORTHY LIFE ACCEPT MY CONGRATULATIONS AND DEEP AFFECTION=

    BISHOP JOHN WESLEY LORD=.

THE COMPANY WILL APPRECIATE SUGGESTIONS FROM ITS PATRONS CONCERNING ITS SERVICE

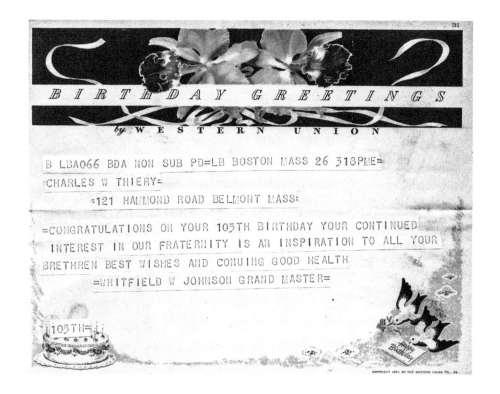

735

BIRTHDAY GREETINGS by WESTERN UNION

B LBA066 BDA NON SUB PD=LB BOSTON MASS 26 318PME=

CHARLES W THIERY=

    =121 HAMMOND ROAD BELMONT MASS=

=CONGRATULATIONS ON YOUR 105TH BIRTHDAY YOUR CONTINUED

INTEREST IN OUR FRATERNITY IS AN INSPIRATION TO ALL YOUR

BRETHREN BEST WISHES AND CONUING GOOD HEALTH

    =WHITFIELD W JOHNSON GRAND MASTER=

105TH

COPYRIGHT 1941 BY THE WESTERN UNION TEL. CO.

John A. Collins, President
Earle M. Prescott, Vice-President

E. Robert Higgs
- EDITOR -

THE BELL

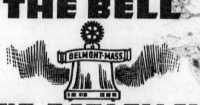

VOL. 24

NO. 17
OCTOBER 26, 1955

BELMONT ROTARY CLUB 2759

"Service above Self" He Profits Most Who Serves Best

That wonderful, young fellow - CHARLES W. THIERY - was with us on Tuesday night to celebrate his ONE HUNDRED FIFTH (105) birthday. His birthday is actually on October 26 and this is the sixth time he has honored us with his presence at birthday time.

EARLE PRESCOTT had the honor of presenting MR. THIERY to the members -- and he got a tremendous rising ovation. As the crowd sang "HAPPY BIRTHDAY," he was presented with a birthday cake — the compliments of WALTER SUTHERLAND — and that well-known chain of bakeries -- DOROTHY MURIEL'S.

AND -- you know what! At the meeting of the Board of Directors - later on in the evening - CHARLIE THIERY was made an HONORARY MEMBER of our Club!! You can all call him "CHARLIE" from now on! We hope that he will avail himself of the privilege of coming to our meetings often.

GIL BALL gave out other birthdays for October:

Stan Russell	10-6	Tot Hoople	10-12
Doc MacLean	10-7	Sid Farrell	10-23
Frank Lally	10-8	Gordon Seavey	10-25
Gibby Gibson	10-10	J. Danahy	10-27

KEN COX introduced the following visitors:

CAMBRIDGE: John Giles....... Ray Chaffee
                Arthur Hydren.. A. J. del'Etoile
                .... Harold A. Ryan, Jr.
BOSTON: Bill Wood .... Ralph Lull
                .... John Marquard
WALTHAM: Manson Dillaway........ Nick
                                    Cannistraro
CONCORD: .... Glenn Simm
MARBLEHEAD: .... Elliott Roundy
ARLINGTON: .... Charles Wyman

GUESTS: - - Walter Anderson - Gibby Gibson
              and Harold Pollock - Earl Allen
HONORARY ROTARIAN: - - - - Ralph Ward
JR. ROTARIANS: - - - - Jonathan Brower and
                            Dudne Breeze

The 68 Members and 18 Visitors enjoyed a beef pie dinner, with green salad, & custard pie or ice cream roll for dessert.

The Absentees were: Anderson; Cooke; Cox, John; Danahy; Donaldson; Flett; Hesseltine; Goddard; Hathaway; Hollis; Johnson; Kunos; Kramer; Olive; Ross; Seavey; Short; Stengel.

We were glad to see BILL WOOD out and he was the first to get the "HONORARY BOO". We understand some other permanent visitors are seeking this honor, but you really have to earn it!

JUDGE ELIAS SHAMAN of the Boston Municipal Court gave us a mighty interesting talk on the Nations of the Near East and how explosive the situation is right now.

PRES. JOHN has a gold pencil which some one has lost. Is it yours?

The ROTARY-ANNS have invited us all to their "Gentlemen's Night" on Nov. 22. Better check with the missus and be ready to make reservations.

NEXT WEEK: HOWARD FOWLER, Editor of the Mansfield News.
SUBJECT: - - "The Country Editor Speaks"

BOB HIGGS,
. EDITOR

WILLIAM F. CLARK
M∴E∴GRAND HIGH PRIEST
660 BELMONT ST., WATERTOWN 72

COMMENDATION
of the
GRAND ROYAL ARCH CHAPTER OF MASSACHUSETTS

Dear Companion:

On this twenty-sixth day of October, A.D. 1950, A.I. 2480, we hail, greet and congratulate you as a Royal Arch Mason worthy of special commendation.

Your unbroken record of continued membership in the Massachusetts Capitular Rite, extending over a period of seventy years, is an enviable one.

We are happy to recognize you as a courtesy to Cambridge Royal Arch Chapter, of which for so many years you have been a member; and we greet you personally in the most sincere bonds of companionship, and congratulate the Chapter in this testimonial to you.

May you and your Chapter continue for many years in that united Service, Love and Loyalty so splendidly reflected in the exceptional record which you have established as one of its members.

In recognition of your splendid achievement, I hereunto set my hand and with it the Seal of this Grand Body.

Companion Charles W. Thiery

Born October 26, 1850   Exalted June 11, 1880

Recognition by Grand Chapter
October 26, 1950

Attest:

William F. Clark
M∴E∴ Grand High Priest

Raymond F. Newall
R∴W∴E∴ Grand Secretary

Chapter 8.

"Work don't kill a man"

"You'll find few men who work as hard as I do"

UNCLE CHARLIE WAS REGULARLY pulled out of school to be a messenger boy for his father's business. The Civil War (1861-1865) was raging during his childhood, and he served as a drummer boy for the Boston Light Dragoons. Uncle Charlie often mentioned he spent his growing up years being outside.

When I was growing up, World War II (U.S., 1941-1945) was raging, as the U. S. became totally engaged in the war effort. Like Uncle Charlie, I was outside when not in school. I just returned each night for supper.

Bill Stone's family market garden and dairy business, a mile from home, was one of my playgrounds. Farmers' sons have daily chores to complete. No childhood friends would be allowed to pull them away from their work. So, I helped out, stripping milk from cows after the milking machines got the bulk of the milk. I drove work-horses pulling harrows, plows, rakes, and wagons. Then, we transitioned to Massey Ferguson tractors, pulling the same implements and wagons. We fed the animals and cultivated the land.

In a newspaper interview with Uncle Charlie it was stated that

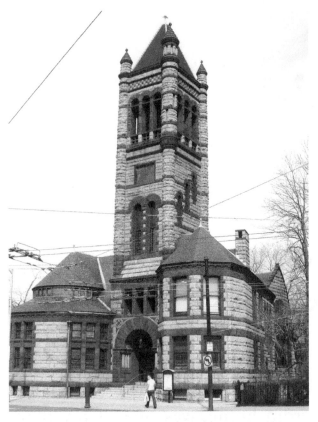

Harvard-Epworth United Methodist Church

"the watch case business 'faded out in the late 1870's'. In 1880 Thiery became a gold buyer, a business he followed until he retired…" According to the supply of gold, his business was active or slow. He adjusted to changes to stay in business. He was involved in jewelry and bookselling when the gold supply was limited.

Uncle Charlie retired in 1943 at age 93. Two years before retirement, his Harvard Street Church merged with Epworth Methodist Church to become the Harvard-Epworth United Methodist Church at a new location where it remains today, 1555 Massachusetts Avenue, Harvard Square in Cambridge.

When Uncle Charlie left his "life outdoors" and started working for his father in the watchcase business, at about age 14, a newspaper article said, "Thiery began having digestive troubles which have plagued him ever since…"

I wasn't pulled out of school but I worked and played outside until sundown when I returned home for supper. Some of my paid work was for Penobscot Mountain Bottling Company, a water and soda bottler; and then a Mobile gas station—pumping gas, changing tires, batteries and doing minor repairs, oil and grease jobs. Other local work was as a soda jerk at a drugstore a few hundred yards from home. We lived about a quarter mile from the public library, which I was paid to clean. My mother, an operating room nurse, came behind me and cleaned up what I didn't see.

In 1875, at age 25, Uncle Charlie went to San Francisco (Berkeley) for 18 months to instruct a company on how to manufacture his family business's proprietary watch case covers.

In the Civil War period, Uncle Charlie joined the 1st Brigade—Cavalry of the Boston Light Dragoons, the Massachusetts state militia. Both of us were age 10 when the wars of our generations began. After eight years he mustered out as a sergeant. Napoleon Bonaparte was Uncle Charlie's hero. A portrait of the French emperor was prominently displayed in his home. Uncle Charlie was asked about Napoleon in an interview. "'Not too many people seem aware of the fact, but Napoleon abhorred war and all of the suffering that went with it.' Thiery said, 'He had his faults, it is true, but no man is perfect. But he was a great man, a truly great man.'" The article stated Uncle Charlie had the largest collection

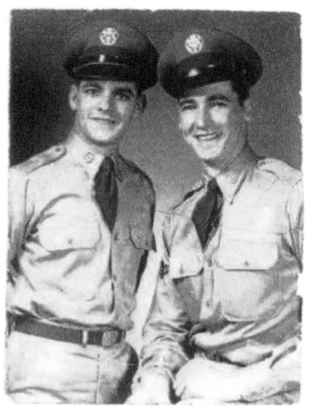

Donald, left, and Joshua

of books about Napoleon in the area.

September, 1950, three months after the outbreak of the Korean War, my twin brother, Donald, and I joined the Air Force. Over the next three decades, I continued on in active reserve duty following active duty, retiring as a Lieutenant Colonel on 20 April 1981 (my 50th birthday). I've always had at least two occupations. Although I've loved pursuing my three passions—flying, selling, and playing with words (writing), you'd probably have to label me a workaholic. Long work days are not easy for spouses to live with. My heavy work schedule likely led to the end of my first marriage after 24 years and four children.

Uncle Charlie had to adapt to the ups and downs of the gold market. The 1896 Alaskan, 1848 Californian, and 1828 Dahlonega, Georgia gold rushes influenced the supply available. Gold "petered out after the 1934 Gold Reserve Act" Uncle Charlie said. This law made it a criminal offense for U.S. citizens to own or trade gold anywhere in the world, with limited exceptions. It was reported, "He left that business because he was cheated so many times, but when he entered it again after requests from his many customers he realized that he had gone through all the frauds and had become an expert."

When not gold dealing, Uncle Charlie was a bookseller and in the jewelry business. Newspaper reporter Alta Maloney wrote,

"Looking back, Thiery is pleased that he has been a success in every business he has tried."

In my case, I graduated in the top 20% of my Air Force Electronics class at age 20 in 1951, and subsequently was a "Distinguished Cadet Graduate" from flight training in 1953.

In 1956, as a full time student at Harvard, I bought my first home and subsequent larger home as a real estate broker. In the spring of my senior year, I sold five upscale homes to supplement my GI Bill funding to pay for college and support a wife and three children. I was spending a lot of money commuting 20 miles to Cambridge and Manchester, New Hampshire, flying short active reserve missions for the Air Force National Guard. Harvard University loaned me money, but would not give me a scholarship due to my earning too much money!

I was either perched in a jet aircraft, sitting in a classroom or library, selling real estate, or commuting back and forth to go where I needed to be.

Graduating in 1959, I spent the next two years successfully managing two Boston suburban residential subdivisions, West Peabody and North Reading, Massachusetts. Working with another salesman, we earned the nickname "the gold dust twins." We took turns being recognized as salesman of the month.

My older brother, John, persuaded me to enter the life insurance business in New York City. In 1961, after less than a year in the Big Apple, my southern wife wanted to return to her home state of Georgia. Moving to Atlanta, I achieved Million Dollar Round Table (MDRT) sales recognition while flying for the Air Force Air National Guard Active Reserve. How was I able to be successful for many years in both occupations at the same time? I sold insurance to fellow airmen.

During our worldwide trips, if asked a question about insurance from a fellow air crew member, I'd promise to call after we returned to our home base. This way, we stayed focused on our Air Force mission and I wouldn't be hounding them while we were on flying duty. I learned that it wasn't professional or productive to sell at inappropriate times.

Now in my fourth quarter of life, I don't plan to retire just like my role model Uncle Charlie. I'm living my third quarter affirmation, to magnify the value of my experiences. Now I'm speaking and writing, as an author, about lessons learned to live long and live well. The insurance business and investments are financing the completion of this, my eighth book.

Chapter 9.

"I've all this money I don't know what to do with."

SPRING OF '54 GRAVESIDE PROPOSAL

THE FIRST QUESTION NEWS reporters and others asked Uncle Charlie was, "To what do you attribute your long life?" He would answer, "I've no wife to scold me and no children to worry me. I don't smoke or drink"; and occasionally with a smile, "I'm a lifelong Republican!" The next questions would be about bachelorhood.

There are many theories that explain why Uncle Charlie remained single. Chapter XI, The Paradox of Perfectionism, poses many reasons. An analytical personality likes to watch others, learn from their mis-

takes, and avoid repeating them. He said to a reporter, "Marriage is all right if you found the right woman, but how would you know before the wedding?" Workaholics like Uncle Charlie are so focused on work that they take little time for the "dating game". He remarked to a reporter he'd begin working Monday morning, "under a strain, and continued under a strain, through the week, as if he were in Napoleon's army in a forced march…at times ending the week at 1:30 AM Sunday morning."

Uncle Charlie lost his mother when he was 15. When he was 20, he lost his sister, Julia, to the same Bright's (kidney) disease.

Throughout the years, Uncle Charlie opened his Bible to get answers. Repeatedly the answer was "no" about "popping the question."

And then, there's stature and demeanor. How many women are chasing 5'3" short dictatorial men?

Uncle Charlie understood the excitement of weddings when on March 29, 1953, he walked my sister, Joan, down the aisle (our father had died seven years before). *The Boston Herald* reporter asked on this occasion, "How does it happen that you never married?" Uncle Charlie said, "I had to stick to business. Father's business was in a precarious state when I went into it."

That left meeting eligibles through work, civic/community meetings, and charitable events. In his time, most organizations were for either men or women, not co-ed.

Houghton Mifflin publishing company founder, Henry Oscar Houghton (b. 30 April 1823), was a member of the Harvard Street Methodist Church. For many years,

he was superintendent of their Sunday school, where Uncle Charlie taught. His daughter was Elizabeth "Lizzie" Harris Houghton. She was named after his "beloved" first wife who died years before Lizzie was born to Nanna Weir (Wyer) Manning, Henry Oscar Houghton's second wife. They were married on 12 September 1854.[1] Uncle Charlie and Lizzie became closer when they worked together managing book sales; and, they had a mutual interest in charitable causes. Note: Cambridge Historical Society Secretary and Author, Albert Harrison Hall, wrote (1916) that Elizabeth Harris Haughton, born 6 March, 1858, was active in the parish work of Christ Church. Lizzie's obituary mentioned both parents were members of Christ Church.

In the year Lizzie was 57 years old (1915) and Uncle was 65, "she died as the result of a distressing automobile accident near Harvard Square on May 20, 1915."[2] My twin brother, Donald, told me that Uncle Charlie

1. Biography of Henry Oscar Houghton, 1897, Horace Scudder. Riverside Press
2. Albert Harrison Hall, Cambridge Historical Society

told him that Lizzie "spurned" him and it was God's punishment to her that she died a week or so later. Sister Nancy often heard Uncle Charlie utter in an animated way, "Lizzie."

This is another instance of Uncle Charlie losing someone he cared about. Medium Tom Flynn, Chapter X, said Uncle Charlie "went to his mother for love." As you have already read, he lost her when he was 15.

Nancy was his beautiful, intelligent, young grandniece; her features favor the Theiry side of our family. We know from Chapter VI that she accompanied him to the 1953 Republican Club Banquet featuring President Dwight "Ike" Eisenhower. Photos of them appeared in a page of photos covering that event in the *Boston Globe* on September 22, 1953. After years of being a celebrated centenarian, was Uncle Charlie enjoying a new sense of importance? My first wife of a few months, Naunie, lived with Nancy in Boston while I was on active duty in Labrador, Canada. Naunie also attended Harvard-Epworth United Methodist Church

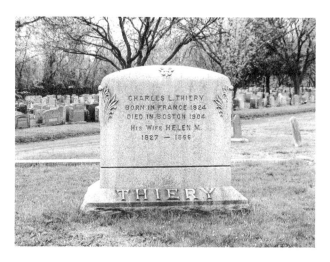

with Uncle Charlie. She saw him as a "cute little man." He was pleased when she quickly found the hymns and psalms in hymnals at the services. Naunie believes he imagined Nancy as a "trophy wife." (Recall the Boston Globe picture of Uncle Charlie and Nancy in Chapter VI). While he wouldn't allow others to hold his arm while ascending stairs, he, as a gentleman, allowed Naunie to do so.

Had he found his Biblical OK when on a spring day in 1954 he asked Nancy to marry him? Nancy's account follows:

"Uncle Charlie asked me to accompany him for a visit to the family plot at the Cambridge Cemetery. We travelled by trolley. Graveside, at the intersection of Tulip Path,

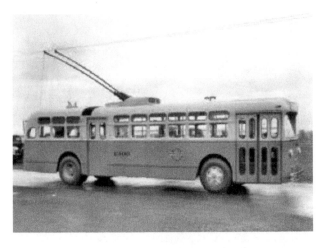

Winchester, and Laurel Avenues, we sat on a big rock overlooking the Thiery family plot. He talked briefly about our deceased family members. I recall that his proposal was very direct, 'I have all this money I'm not sure what to do with.' Dumbfounded, I could only blurt out, 'But we're related, but we're related!' Awkward silence followed. We returned to his residence on the trolley.

By the time I had travelled back 20 miles to my home in Sudbury, Frank Merritt, Uncle Charlie's landlord and close friend, had already chastised Uncle Charlie. Frank called my mother on behalf of Uncle Charlie and apologized." Reflecting on this whole event, one can see a number of good and sufficient reasons for Uncle Charlie's last stand (like Custer's) for a close personal relationship.

It's clear Uncle Charlie knew what to do with all his money. In 1952, Uncle Charlie completed a very detailed will. It laid out many bequests for worthy causes including his church, family, and friends. This leads to another scenario. Uncle Charlie witnessed Nancy helping our nurse mother deal with her broken leg and two senior patients. Nancy was scurrying about, shopping and serving during our mother's recovery. Uncle Charlie was aware of her caring dedication. Also, Nancy noted that following the failed graveside proposal, there was a codicil to Uncle Charlie's will. It seems possible that Uncle Charlie concluded that since Nancy did not agree to be his wife, that left him relying, for his personal care, on his landlord and landlady, the Merritts. He changed his bequest to the Merritts from $25 a week to a single lump sum of $5,000. Mr and Mrs Merritt had failing health. The natural

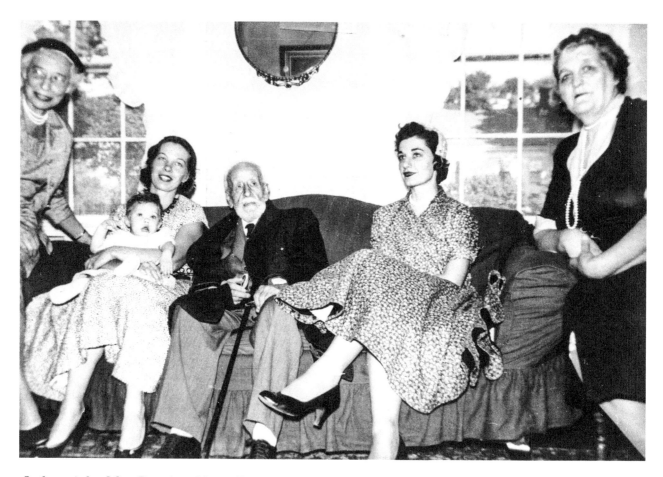

Left to right, Mrs. Bunting, Nancy Bunting Batchelder and baby Janie, Uncle Charlie, Nancy Elizabeth Batchelder and Mother Emma Macaulay Batchelder October 1955.

question, who will take care of me when they're gone? Could Uncle Charlie's money buy him help for the rest of his life? Nancy would then have become his comfortable caregiver.

See the picture above, taken a year later, at Uncle Charlie's 105th birthday family celebration. Their body language tells us Uncle Charlie and Nancy remained guarded. She was on her way to South Af-

rica for work for the State Department.

In 1956, a UPI news article, *Life of a Bachelor, Good for 106 Years,* Belmont, Massachusetts, Uncle Charlie celebrated his 106th birthday "toasting the woman he never found."

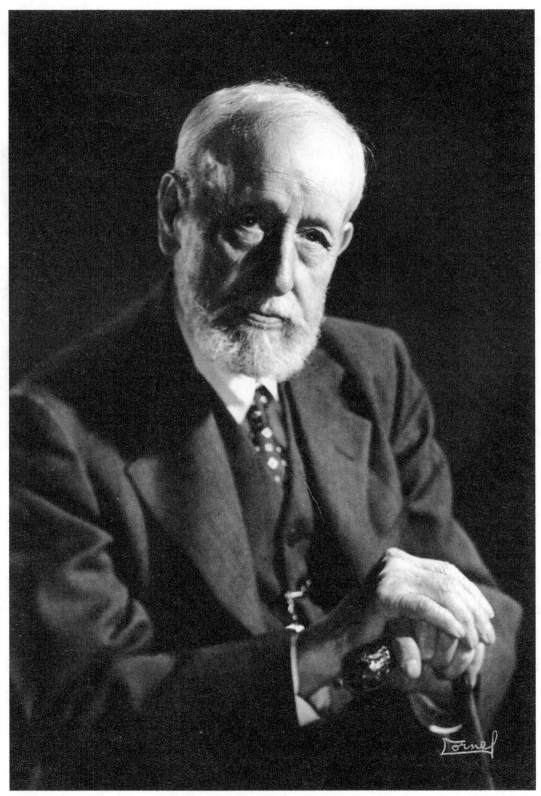

Wise and witty Uncle Charlie at 103

Chapter 10.
Finishing Touches
THE LEGEND SPEAKS FROM BEYOND, 16 MAY 2013

EARLY MAY 2012, I traveled to Wellesley, Massachusetts, to collect a scrapbook covering Uncle Charlie. My father's sister, Marie Batchelder Tufts, a niece of Uncle Charlie's, had maintained it. Her daughter, my cousin, Doris, gave it to me. It is a treasure trove. It is filled with pictures, stories, letters, and telegrams related to Uncle Charlie's last seven and one half years of life (26 October, 1950 until 16 March, 1958).

With this rich accumulation of material, especially all of Uncle Charlie's answers to news reporters' questions and family memories, I sought to learn more about his personal, work, and family life.

The content of letters written at age 106 in addition to handwriting analysis of his writing strokes told me more about his personality traits. This information was especially helpful for evaluating all the stories about his personal habits, opinions, and values. However, these efforts only prompted more questions, including documentation to support Uncle Charlie's service in the Massachusetts State Militia Cavalry, charitable work, and personal connections. Remember, my sister Nancy recalled Uncle Charlie often muttering the name "Lizzie"; and my twin brother Donald, also close to Uncle Charlie, especially in his later years, told of his involvement with Lizzie Houghton earlier in his life. A week after Lizzie "spurned" Uncle Charlie, she died in a tragic car accident in Harvard Square (20 May, 1915). Uncle Charlie told Donald he believed it was "God's punishment." From Nancy and Donald's recollections I researched and discovered that Lizzie was one Elizabeth Harris Houghton, born 6 March 1858, eight years after Uncle Charlie. The Cambridge Historical Society identifies Lizzie as the daughter of Henry Oscar Houghton, founder of the Houghton Mifflin Publishing Company. Remembering that Uncle Charlie was a bookseller after the family watch case making business failed, I surmised that Uncle Charlie knew Henry Oscar Houghton through their mutual Methodist Church memberships. A college classmate of Henry Oscar, Horace E. Scudder, wrote his biography, *Henry Oscar Houghton A Biographical Outline* (1897). This book reveals that Henry Oscar was the superintendent of the Harvard Street Methodist Church Sunday school. Uncle Charlie, 27 years Henry Oscar's junior, taught Sunday school there for three decades. I concluded Uncle Charlie likely became a bookseller through his church connection with Henry Oscar. The Cambridge Historical Society led me to conclude that Lizzie was very active in Christ Church, Harvard Square, Cambridge. Her obituary confirms that her parents were active members of the same Christ Church. Lizzie was also involved with many charitable causes beyond Christ Church. Uncle Charlie's will proves that he actively supported many charities in their community, where he and Lizzie shared an ongoing relationship in addition to their bookselling connection. Lizzie's 1910 last will and testament is evidence of her strong devotion to family, friends, and charitable causes.

Searching for more clues and missing evidence, I turned to a source many detectives try – a psychic. Note: My life experiences have helped me conclude that one should not spend a lot of time, money and hang their hat on readings, i.e., having a blind faith on what can be gained from consulting a medium. Still, it's usually a sliver or two of information that can prove very helpful. My mother, Emma B. Macaulay Batchelder, was an operating room nurse. She often told me of near death experiences (NDE) and the "wonders of the spirit world" her patients revealed. I had a twenty-four year marriage to a gifted psychic, my first wife.

I've read about Duke University research headed by psychologist J. B. Rhine that explored ESP (Extrasensory Perception). Dr. Rhine was committed to scientific examination of ESP findings and exposing fraud. A 1980 book, *The Airmen Who Would Not Die*, by John Grant Fuller, Jr., recounts how Duke University and British Psychic Society researchers had a unique opportunity to study psychic work done by Eileen Garrett, a famous Irish medium, regarding the crash of a dirigible (airship) on 5 October 1930 in France.

In a situation similar to the US Space Shuttle Challenger mission, engineers of the British R101 Airship had said it was not ready for a round trip mission to India which would have been a world first – its maiden overseas voyage. On a windy, rainy day it took off from England, crossed over the English Channel only to crash in France.

Before any crash investigation was mounted, Eileen Garrett had connected many of the victims of the tragedy and their families. Eileen could not have known in advance the highly technical engineering information she was relaying. Evidence was recovered by this method without any detectable fraud.

In Uncle Charlie's own family, a murder weapon was located under the direction of a medium, who visualized it behind a staircase. It fingered the murderer.

In Mid-May of 2013, I traveled to Berkeley, California, to consult a widely known English medium, Tom Flynn. Tom can neither read nor write. The following information was relayed to me without prompting. I was looking for more evidence to reconstruct Uncle Charlie's life.

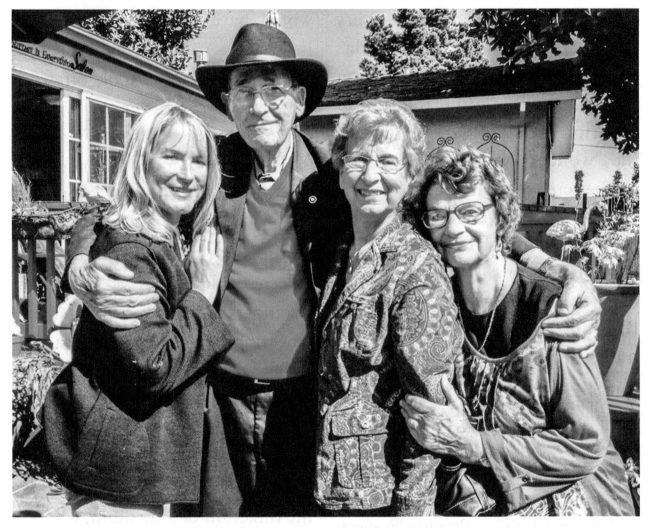

Left to right: Karen, Josh, wife Betty Ann, and sister Nancy at the patio
when the consultation with Tom Flynn took place.

1. Uncle Charlie went fast at the end. The "old man's friend," pneumonia, took him.

2. He had a "banging, uneven heart." One news story about Uncle Charlie stated he had survived a heart attack and would afterwards stop at staircase landings to catch his breath.

3. Uncle Charlie's connection with the Houghtons, book selling for Henry Oscar and charitable work with Lizzie, was for a much longer duration than I would have guessed.

4. I asked Tom about Uncle Charlie's time working with Lizzie and the nature of their relationship. "He (Uncle Charlie) got emotion-

al, saying 'It would have been a marriage of convenience, that and nothing more.' His dream was with someone else. He 'watched over and guided Lizzie for many years.'" She was eight years younger than Uncle Charlie. This was an answer to my question regarding Uncle Charlie's time in the bookselling business. "Uncle Charlie said he was in 'a forced situation with Lizzie.' Henry Oscar Houghton died in 1895 when Uncle Charlie was 45 years old. Uncle Charlie's and Lizzie's charitable work could have easily kept them close for years after that."

5. Tom said Uncle Charlie was a great listener and looked carefully before he jumped into a situation. Note: This fits well with his perfectionist, analytical, sometimes procrastinating ways indicated by his handwriting strokes (see Chapter II).

6. He loved music, especially soft tones. I thought of his being a drummer boy with the 1st Brigade of the Boston Light Dragoons during the Civil War period. He saw himself as being in a "forced march" throughout his daily work life, as if he were in Napoleon's army. Did Uncle Charlie actively reflect that steady drum beat throughout his life? He chose the music for his church's commemorative service recognizing his 100th birthday celebration.

7. Regarding missing documents, Tom indicated Uncle Charlie said everything was taken from him at the end of his life and someone misplaced his military papers.

8. "Uncle Charlie was always a very determined man." Note: This is an extra strong dominate trait that can be seen clearly in his handwriting, look at his extended straight down strokes without loops on the letter Y.

9. Tom said it would not be easy for someone to copy Uncle Charlie's business success and other achievements. This is definitely true as Uncle Charlie died a rich man. As reported in a news article, he was "pleased he was a success in every

business he tried. He dealt with the pubic excellently bookselling."

10. Uncle Charlie would consult the Bible about solving his problems. He'd open the book and "get so much wisdom from it." This was often stated in news reports. Tom saw Uncle Charlie holding back tears as he reported he wasn't so sure about finding the answers there for his own personal life. Uncle Charlie went to his mother for love. I concluded losing her when he was 15 and his sister at 20 deeply affected him.

11. Tom reported that a cousin "with black hair" has Uncle Charlie's trunk and Bible. Part of my May 2013 trip was dedicated to locating these items. Unquestionably, it was my cousin Doris (approaching 90 years of age), who has black hair. She has no recollection of possessing them, or their whereabouts. Uncle Charlie said they're still there, as are other items included in his will.

12. Uncle Charlie had a secretive, loner side to his personality. Downward handwriting y-strokes without loops are associated with introversion. Through Tom I learned, "He only let certain people into his life." I was one of them. "He loved me listening to his stories, and he tipped his hat to me."

13. Uncle Charlie said he'd shut the door on people if he knew he was right. This is indicated by sharply down slanted T-bars, stiff T-legs and extended straight Y downstrokes in his handwriting.

14. Uncle Charlie was still building his businesses (investments) to the very end. This fits with his marriage proposal to Nancy during the spring of 1954. Uncle Charlie said, "It (their relationship) was definitely in-the-cards." I remember father telling about family members persuading Uncle Charlie to accompany them on a trip to his bank, The Harvard Trust Company, to hear their proposal to take over "the burden" of managing his financial assets during his later years. The story

goes he listened to their take over plans that needed his approval, and said something like this: "Thank you for caring about me. I've done pretty well so far on my own, and I believe I'll continue on the same way." He got up, put on his derby hat, said good day and marched out the door.

15. Tom says, "He was truly a gentleman; and so are you. Uncle Charlie hopes writing about him will keep his name alive."

16. He liked to be with himself. His cursive personal pronoun I (PPI's) is unusual. They are wrapped up in his ending stroke, curling back into his PPI.

17. From Horace Scudder's biography of Henry Oscar Houghton, it's mentioned that Henry Oscar attended both Harvard Street Methodist and Christ Church in Harvard Square. Both souls (Uncle Charlie and Henry Oscar) are encouraging the completion of this book!

18. Uncle Charlie was a happy man. This is indicated in his handwriting by the upward slope of his baselines. Even at age of 106, he had an optimistic view of life.

19. "He liked his free time when he could find it." His numerous statements about "Hard work don't kill a man", his habit of working until 1:30 AM Sunday morning to end the work week, and his perfectionist personality as indicated by his handwriting define him as a workaholic.

20. Uncle Charlie laughed along with Tom and me as he agreed that working for a family business is more stressful than anything else. He was inspired by working for his father, although they often clashed.

21. About my father and Uncle Charlie: "There was nothing they wouldn't do for one another."

22. There were times when Uncle Charlie relied on Lizzie.

23. My attorney father advised Lizzie. "She had problems with others

coming and going." Here's a mystery I'd love to explore further.

24. Uncle Charlie is "not happy" with the recipient of his extensive collection of military books featuring Napoleon. There's been "some mischief."

25. Regarding working with his father in the watchcase business from his early youth, "He was energized working for father, got wisdom from father, but they clashed." This fits with news reports that state Uncle Charlie's stomach problems began when he came in "from the outside" to work for his father around age 14.

Chapter 11.

The Paradox of Perfectionism

EVALUATING UNCLE CHARLIE'S LIFE BY EILEEN PAGE, MASTER GRAPHOANALYST

A PLETHORA OF PICTURES, facts, quotes, behavior, and stories from many sources about Uncle Charlie have been presented. It's time to hear from a professional evaluator, Master Graphoanalyst Eileen Page, MGA. Eileen, my colleague, has special experience with centenarians. The longer a person writes, the more authentic is the expression of their true personality. Letters Uncle Charlie wrote to Emma Batchelder (my mother) and sister Nancy (his grandniece) at age 106 give us ideal samples to examine.

The complexity of Uncle Charlie's personality and Eileen's years of studying perfectionists makes her the best person to deliver the curtain call summary about him.

HANDWRITING ANALYSIS: CHARLES WESLEY THIERY A.K.A. "GREAT UNCLE CHARLIE"

This report has been done according to the principles of Graphoanalysis and does not reflect the opinions of the writer.

Submitted by: Eileen M. Page MA, MGA, www.pageink.net, August, 2012

EVALUATION

Charles Wesley Thiery, a.k.a. "Great Uncle Charlie" can clearly identify with both titles since each has its own unique and perhaps even conflicting characteristics. On one hand, the very formal and upstanding Charles Wesley Thiery represented traditional beliefs in God and country, Yankee frugality, and maintained strong moral convictions. On the other hand, "Great Uncle Charlie" was a warm-hearted, congenial, fun-loving, and generous man. So then, who is the authentic personality? The answer...both are! As I read through the various news articles and studied his handwriting, I realized that he was a very complex man who led quite a simplistic, yet interesting life.

His simplistic life consisted of staying single and having clearly defined belief systems, feelings towards which Charles Wesley Thiery did not ever waver. These beliefs included, the importance of being a Republican and serving your country, never drinking or smoking, working hard, and last but definitely not least, doing what the Bible says. There were no gray areas surrounding these convictions, no room for discussion. He lived his life both personally and professionally emphasizing and implementing their significance.

The complexities of the man is that, in spite of the disciplined mindset that he continuously maintained, Great Uncle Charlie appeared to have enjoyed life and liked to attend social gatherings. It was said of him that, "He spoke easily and wittingly and with a cheerful twinkle in his eye." His writing showed him to be kind, considerate, and generous. He had a sense of style and self-confidence about who he was and I can only imagine that others would admire and appreciate these attributes when in his company.

Over the years, especially when Great Uncle Charlie became a centenarian, one major inquiry was continually repeated. What is your secret to a long life? Most of the time he would answer that it was because he was a bachelor. Once, however, he changed his tune a little and said by the Grace of God and then added that he didn't think his being a bachelor was responsible for his longevity. I guess we will never know for sure, just as perhaps even Great Uncle Charlie didn't know for sure if his being a bachelor mattered.

The many dimensions of Charles Wesley Thiery will be explored in this report. As you learn about this intriguing man through his handwriting, keep in mind the aspects of his personality that may have contributed to his longevity, health issues, business success, and his either having to or maybe even wanting to remain single all 107 years of his life.

PERSONAL AND PROFESSIONAL IDENTITY

The signature represents one's public self; the text represents one's private self. Mr. Thiery's signature is similar in style but is somewhat larger than the writing seen in his text. This difference means that he was able to adapt to social settings and behave in a more outgoing and gregarious way for short periods of time, but that he also had a more prevalent preference for silence and solitude. This is another demonstration of his personality dichotomy.

The flourishes in his signature represent showmanship, a creative flare as well as a desire for attention. The very long exaggerated umbrella-shaped cover stroke over his surname shows a need to have control over and protect his family name. Perhaps his pride was activated so as to uphold the integrity of his ancestry. His signature supports this because it demonstrates that maintaining appearances was important.

I don't feel in any condition to write, nor do I feel in any condition for any thing. Perhaps you will be able to understand it when you reach the age of 106. But I must write as I write not get any letters from you and that would be too bad for I remember I was reading of you traveling in Europe, Asia and Africa and of course I desire to receive, or hear about it all from you. But I

Charles M. Tiffany

There is certainly the presence of his ego in his signature, a trait which made him think that he was right all the time...something that may not be well received in a relationship. The little circle in the beginning of the capital T in his surname represents a jealousy loop. This trait is an asset professionally because it creates a sense of competition to want to get ahead.

Personally, the trait of jealousy is a liability because it can cause the person to become controlling...another potential challenge to establishing a long term relationship. The long straight ending that goes below the baseline in the lower case "y" is the loner stroke....another indicator that he liked to do things his way without consulting others. It also represents an inner determination to finish whatever he sets out to do.

His proper pronoun I also sheds some light on his identity. It is made with a simple back stroke and then gets very complicated as it winds around itself at the top of the letter. Once again, we can see the symbolic representation of the 2 aspects of his personality. Even though he spent most of his years in America, he also could have a little leftover influence from his French, English, and German heritage which he decided to hold onto because he felt it important for him to do so.

As you globally scan the handwriting in the text sample, it is easy to recognize the amazing consistency and rhythm, especially for a man of 106. The passage even speaks of not feeling in any condition to write and yet he had a sense of obligation to correspond since he worried that he would not hear from his niece, Nancy, unless he wrote to her. His sense of responsibility to do the right thing and the kind and caring side to his personality is evident in the forward slant of his writing which means he leads with his heart and emotionally has a desire to reach out to others. This reaching out to others is also confirmed by his cursive writing style in which all the letters are symbolically, "holding hands."

EMOTIONAL RESPONSIVENESS AND ATTITUDE

Great Uncle Charlie's handwriting shows him to be capable of empathy and attunement towards other's needs. What he did was genuinely heartfelt and could show great compassion when the need arose. The downside to this was that he also had so many control traits in his writing that I'm not sure he allowed himself the luxury of showing these emotions as often as he could have. This meant that he had to work overtime keeping all these heartfelt emotions in check. The stress that this effort could have ultimately caused him might account for some of the chronic stomach ailments that he had from childhood. He once mentioned that the strain of taking on more responsibility affected his nervous system and caused him to have attacks of indigestion and sleepless nights. The optimism that is seen in the uphill climb of the baseline of his writing came to light when he told a reporter that the fact he had problems with his health since a young child may have helped with his longevity because it made him take good care of himself and watch what he ate.

While Great Uncle Charlie paid attention to his physical well-being, his emotional well-being seemed to be put on the back burner. The conflict caused between his desire to emote and his need to contain his emotions was probably more responsible for his stomach ailments than just what he ate. The other residual effect of having to contain his emotions is that eventually these stored feelings can be expressed as impulsive overreactions. Perhaps there were more incidences of these overreactions in his early years because he mentioned his mischievous

childhood before age 16 at which time he joined the Harvard Street Methodist Church and reformed his ways.

Nonetheless, even in adulthood, he remained emotionally invested in what he believed. He was known to, on occasion; let his passions get the best of him, which resulted in unpredictable outbursts, usually caused by wanting to make right what he deemed to be wrong. An incident comes to mind when he pulled a cigarette out of a man's mouth and threw it on the ground because he believed smoking was bad.

Work Ethic

One thing about which there is no doubt is the work ethic of Charles Wesley Thiery. From age 11 to 92 he worked primarily in the watch case making business of his father and then went into gold refining. He was known for saying such things as, "Hard work is no killer," and "You'll find few men who work as hard as I do." He was known for going into work early in the morning and staying long into the night…a lifestyle that does not seem to lend itself to one's physical well-being and/or building a long and happy relationship. In fact, when asked by a reporter why he never married he once replied that, "I had to stick to business. Father's business was in a precarious state when I went into it."

His handwriting traits back up this aspect of his personality. His pride and dignity forced him to set high standards and ensured that he would do more than was expected of him. His seemingly medium to heavy pressure gave him the stamina and perseverance to work those long hours. It also added to the strength of his convictions. His advice to modern businessmen was to, "Always follow Christian principles… on that principle and no other did I do business all my life."

Because he was a man of such indelible convictions, a major one being his love of tradition, he would resist change unless it was his idea. In spite of being a religious advocate and being a Sunday school teacher for 30 years, the depth of his writing would have made it difficult for him to forgive and forget. He could potentially hold a grudge for long periods. It would have been his way or the highway. Perhaps this is another good reason why he preferred to work and even live alone. These traits would have made sustaining a relationship very challenging unless he found someone who was willing to let him have his way…all the time.

Mr. Thiery's writing shows that he could be a fair yet a tough taskmaster. His impatience would be tested by incompetence and indolence. He was a team player to some extent and yet was also very self-directed and goal oriented. These traits would potentially manifest as a strong, capable, and confident leader. The strong, straight, and downward slanting t-bars as shown in the following writing sample illustrates that he was a force to be reckoned with.

The significance of these t-bars is enhanced when they are combined with his stubbornness and the fact that he liked…no loved… to be in charge. An example of this would be

ailing for some time but would not give
up until at last he had too and went
the Cambridge Hospital. Well, I suppose
Donald has told you all about it so
I might just say that he is now at home
for a few days just to build up preparatory
to the operation. He could not do that at the
hospital. I don't know how long it will take
for that but he is quite comfortable here so he

how he not only selected the hymns to be sung at his 100th birthday celebration at his church but also selected the topic for the sermon that the minister would give. The title he chose was, "I'm Not Ashamed of the Gospel."

Perhaps this authoritarian rite of passage stemmed from the fact that he became a corporal in the State Cavalry at only 17. In an interview he stated, "If I had my way, I would have every young man and woman get into the military where they would learn discipline, be taught to obey orders and concentrate their minds on their jobs."

MENTAL ACUITY AND ABILITY

One of Mr. Thiery's most powerful assets was his mind. He had the ability to analyze a problem from all angles and come up with a viable solution. He also preferred to discover the solution by himself; he would not be one to ask for help. His thinking could shift gears at a moment's notice and work from his gut instincts if needed. He would also decide to quickly assess information and skim over what he thought to be irrelevant to his needs. His fluidity of thought and oral and written expression probably got him out of a lot of tough spots. One conflict that could be a detriment to him would be that he could sometimes drag his feet, so to speak, and procrastinate to the point that he would have to work under an emergency deadline. However, with his mental acuity, and strong ability to concentrate and block out distractions, it wouldn't surprise me if he was actually able to meet any deadlines that were set.

This emergency deadline situation could arise due to the fact that Great Uncle Charlie was a perfectionist. You might hear him say, "Do it right or don't do it at all." Consequently, if he didn't have the time to do what needed to get done perfectly, he would postpone doing it altogether. Other traits in his handwriting that affirm his perfectionism is his organization ability; attention to detail, consistent and steady rhythm and as contrary as this may seem... his indecisiveness. Indecisiveness is often evident in a perfectionist's writing because once a decision is made, accountability for that decision follows. This can be a stressor for a perfectionist. However, the positive interpretation of this trait is that it leads the person to do a lot of checking and exploration in order to reduce the margin for error. The previously mentioned traits of Great Uncle Charlie dragging his feet and procrastinating can contribute to limiting errors because he could have used that time to research solutions to any problems that he thought might arise.

FEARS AND DEFENSES

Fears in the personality can be very helpful. In moderation they act as motivators to do well; however, in an extreme they are considered counterproductive and sometimes even destructive if there are too many of them. Fortunately, most of the fears seen in Mr. Thiery's handwriting are in the moderate range. His desire for attention that is seen in his signature meant that he did not want to be ignored. The jealousy stroke, also previously mentioned in his signature, meant that he viewed love as a competition and feared that he might lose. This trait, combined with the fear of rejection, leads me to believe that he might have experienced a rejection by someone he cared about and that experience potentially set the tone for his staying single. The fear of rejection limits one's ability to trust in others.

The indecisiveness that is evident in his writing represents a fear of accountability. As already mentioned, this trait is connected to Charlie being a perfectionist and is rooted in the fear of never feeling good enough. In spite of Charlie's continued successes, he might always have had a haunting feeling that he could have done better. That unsettling feeling might also have accounted for the stern and overly disciplining side of his personality.

One of the other fears that Great Uncle Charlie had was a fear of want. Once again we see how his success as a business man was thwarted by the thought he might lose it all. Perhaps his living through the depression kept that fear in the forefront of his mind and also contributed to his conservative lifestyle and Yankee frugality. Because of this, his gener-osity was possibly tempered by selectivity, carefully chosen causes to support. They may have been causes that brought him something in return by way of status or recognition of some sort. This also would fulfill his need for attention.

To counter these fears, we all develop some defenses. Great Uncle Charlie's defenses seemed to be in abundance. It makes me wonder if he lived his life with the concepts of, "Murphy's Law." He seemed to have every angle covered with a plan in place just in case something didn't go as expected. One of Charlie's healthier adjustment defenses evident in his handwriting was caution in his day to day decision making. He was a risk-taker, but a very conservative one. Other adjustment defenses included his dry sense of humor, intuitiveness, reticence, poise, and loyalty, all of which I'm sure served him well in social situations.

Great Uncle Charlie also had many resistant defenses from which to choose, and was ready to take on whatever or whoever challenged him. His writing showed that he liked a spirited debate and an opportunity to let someone know what he thought. The downside to this is that his writing also illustrates that he was not very receptive about hearing another's ideas, especially those that were contrary to his own. He was so passionately invested in his beliefs that it would be very difficult, if not impossible, to ever change his mind.

He was a man who was very set in his ways, a creature of habit, and staying single allowed him to do what he wanted and when he wanted to do it. These "fight defenses" as they are sometimes referred to, represent a resistance to change and would have been a hindrance to sustaining a relationship that would potentially require any attitude adjustments on his part and ultimately his lifestyle.

CONCLUSION

Charles Wesley Theiry left quite a legacy behind; one that appears to be much bigger than his 5 foot, 3 inch frame would imply. Those that met him well after his 100th birthday were still duly impressed with his firm handclasp and the appearance of his strong, sturdy looking body and brisk gait. Doctors studied him to learn how he managed to get to his age and still have good eyesight (he only wore reading lenses), fair to good hearing, with many of his mental faculties still functioning so effectively. Perhaps this was due in part to the fact that he walked every day... sometimes for hours. Getting to know Charles through this endeavor, I can't help but think that staying single was a contributing factor also.

It has been an interesting and rewarding adventure getting to know Charles Wesley Theiry and his alter ego, Great Uncle Charlie. I have developed a great respect for his courage and stamina to do all that he accomplished, and I envy his longevity.

Great Uncle Charlie was a survivor. He did what he thought was best to get through life in a way that was comfortable for him...and that strategy certainly seemed to work well for him. Whether that lifestyle would have been one that a, "significant other" would have learned to value as much as he did remains a question.

And so for the reader, I present these questions. After becoming acquainted with the various descriptions of Great Uncle Charlie's personality and after exploring some of the many dimensions of his life's journey, what do you think accounted for his longevity? Why do you think he remained a bachelor all his life? Do you think it was a conscious choice not to marry, or was it because he could never find that perfect person to complement his personality?

Only Charles Wesley Thiery a.k.a. Great Uncle Charlie knows for sure.

May he rest in peace.

Chapter 12.
Living Long and Living Well
THE 100 PLUS CLUB

IF YOU HAVE A mindset of 100 plus years of life, you'll take on more challenges without the fear of running out of time.

I was approaching forty, with many mid-life challenges, as my insurance business focus and connections were changing. At 6'3" I was nearing 260 pounds. My blood pressure was at the high end of the normal range, and I was falling asleep on the couch at the end of stressful work days. My active reserve duty service—flying around the world navigating military transport aircraft—was nearing its end. My attempts at different types of physical exercise weren't taking. Jogging, for example. I just didn't like it. Isometrics wasn't difficult, but it bored me. Weight lifting didn't appeal to me because I wasn't reaching for big muscles. What appealed to me was hatha yoga – its philosophy and promises. I read *Yoga, Youth and Reincarnation* by Jess Stearn. As a skeptical New York City journalist, he traveled to a Concord, Massachusetts, ashram and discovered the immediate physical, mental, and emotional benefits from practicing the hatha yoga discipline.

During 1970-71, I took nine months of weekly training under the tutelage of a master yoga guru. Shortly after, I found a second teacher, Tim Geoghegan. He was an Irish wrestler who became a physical therapist. My yoga regimen led to more energy and endurance at age forty than I recall having at age twenty-two.

On July 26, 1972, our fourth child, Rebecca, arrived, fourteen years after our third child. I could run with her, climb Stone Mountain, and carry her back down the mountain when she sprained her ankle.

A second book I read about yoga, *Be Young with Yoga* (7th printing, 1971). The author was the famous TV instructor, Richard Hittleman. It includes a seven week course that is a clear plan to maintain vitality for a more productive life. My new exercise routine helped me manage the stress involved with selling insurance. A second wind gave me three hours more productive evening time. No longer would the family watch me fall asleep on the couch in front of the TV.

Subsequently, I added the power and unique advantages of rebounding exercise with music. Astronauts use rebounders for balance and aerobic benefits. It delivers negative G-forces, not possible to achieve with most other exercise programs.

The aerobic benefits of rebounding are clearly experienced at the twelve minute point when you become aware of the increased blood flow. It's the same as the euphoria you get when jogging. Once the euphoria kicks in, it's easier to keep on running. Playing rhythmic music adds pleasure to this activity. Because rebounding is so dynamic, beginners should seek guidance and understanding to avoid damaging their bodies. You achieve the full benefits in twenty to twenty-five minutes without the time demands of other exercise programs.

On 20 April 1981, I retired from active reserve flying duty. This gave me time for new activities. I still continued my work in aerospace education as a volunteer with the Georgia Wing Staff of the Civil Air Patrol. It was during this new phase of life that I helped found and give a name to The 100 Plus Club. Through my insurance business and other interests, I helped assemble a group of like-minded professionals. We researched the varied systems, equipment, and skills needed for the longevity clinics we envisioned. The players were as follows:

Jim Mitchell, Manager at Control Data Corporation. Jim was our healed basketball star who introduced Fred Allman, MD, to the group.

Don Kammer, Engineer/Designer of Medical Equipment, was a WWII Fighter Pilot, gymnast, and engineer and 32 year business owner with Lybron Flarshein & Ritter. He was our outreach to the medical profession.

Fred Sliman, Nutronics, coordinated our scientific measurement of members; that is, their metabolic performance and needs. He also served medical professionals.

Clark Cameron, PhD, Psychologist, was our chief inventor, architect and coordinator of the systems and psychology for assessing the mental aspects of member behavior modification.

Margaret Williamson, Registered Dietician, with a Master's in Public Health. She had a high position with the State of Georgia in Public Health.

Ann Worachak, also a registered dietician, was to coordinate, train and direct our effort to provide individualized programs that relate nutrition to life style analysis. They will qualify and amplify Fred Sliman's Nutronics report.

Sandra Jones, RN, and Louis Leonardi, Professional Athlete, were professionally trained, certified, and experienced by operating an existing health clinic. Louis is a former track star. They were to coordinate, train, and supervise the "people flow" and good handling of our first clinic.

Fred Allman, MD, Orthopedic Medicine, owner of Atlanta Sports Medicine.

Lastly, myself, CGA, CLU, ChFC, U.S. Air Force, Lt. Colonel, (Retired), the Chief Wing Navigator, salesman, and motivator who will add career cultivation and quality of life issues to help people – our members – to live long and live well.

Dr. Clark Cameron outlined the design for The 100 Plus Club and Longevity Clinics (see paper, attached).

Getting members to stick with their programs through behavior modification was viewed as essential. Dr. Allman stated this was the key to real success of longevity clinics.

After a year of meetings, we didn't raise the money needed for our start-up, and personal and/or business demands caused us to disband. Still, individually we all gained from our efforts.

Five Subconscious Programs Essential to Success

By Clark T. Cameron, PhD, Sales Psychologist for The 100 Plus Club

As used here, the concept of "success" refers to the attainment of goals that are subconsciously selected and sought. At the subconscious level, of course, people succeed automatically and unconsciously at carrying out their programming, regardless of the consequences, until their doing so results in sufficient frustrations or trauma that they reprogram.

In varying degrees, most human beings are equipped with one or more of the basic success programs outlined below. Some people experience all of them almost all the time, in all of life's areas of challenge and reward. Others experience them only in regard to one area, such as business or family life, or experience only one of the programs.

Research has shown that each person's subconscious mind has perfect knowledge of each of these programs, precisely how effective it is, and under exactly which conditions it is operational; precisely what causes brought it into being, and what penalties it exacts.

Research has also demonstrated that each of these programs, even if presently non-existent, or only fractionally effective for any years or an entire lifetime, is readily and rapidly capable of being changed and of being brought to the 100% effective level. The first in this process is removal of the corresponding Five

Deadly Subconscious Obstacles to Success.

Finally, research has demonstrated that the subconscious information governing these programs may be readily accessed and brought to the conscience level for review and action by using the Cheek-LeCron method. Desired changes may then be rapidly produced using some or all of the various SGS approaches and methods.

1. Basic Success Program. I'm destined to succeed, I can't help succeeding, I always succeed, I automatically succeed, I will succeed, I am succeeding, I am a success, etc.

2. Dislike of Failure Program. I dislike failing, I hate failure, I refuse to fail, I never fail, I am not a failure, failure is not my thing, I despise failing, etc. Note: Modern Psychology would drop this dislike of failure program.

3. Love of Success Program. I deserve to succeed, I love success, I love winning, I love being a success, success feels great, success really turns me on, I'm happy with success, I love winning, I love to be on top, I am in love with winning, etc.

4. Full Permission to Succeed. It's absolutely OK for me to succeed, everyone allows me to succeed, it's absolutely right for me to be a success, I'm doing the right things being successful, it's great for me to get ahead of others by winning, it's wonderful for me to beat out other people in competitions, I've got a complete go-ahead in succeeding, when I win, everyone wins, my parents love me to succeed, my spouse loves me to be successful, etc.

5. I Can Handle Success Program. I can handle success, I have everything I need to cope with great success, whenever I'm successful, I know just what to do next, things work out fine for me when I'm successful, when I'm successful everything in my life goes right, the more successful I am the happier and healthier I am, the more friends I have, the better my life is, etc.

Note: At this moment, using the Cheek-LeCron method, each person's subconscious mind is capable, within minutes, of reporting to the conscience level, on a 0—100 scale, the exact extent to which it is now programmed with each and every one of the five programs above.

ᏕᏕᏕ SUCCESS GUIDANCE SYSTEMS, inc.

THE ONE HUNDRED PLUS CLUB AND LONGEVITY CLINICS

Science has now provided simple, effective methods, disciplines and equipment that can make it possible for the average person, who decides to do so, to live many decades past the century mark in vigorous good health of body and mind.

There are three major areas of relatively recent discovery which-- in the context of modern medical and health sciences-- play the key role in enabling people to produce this significant breakthrough in human life expectancy:

(1) Psychology. People program their own death ages and methods into their subconscious minds. Using remarkable new methods discovered by medical hypnotherapists, they may now ascertain what these ages and methods are, and then change them. On a continuing basis, other psychological stressing forces that debilitate or destroy the body may also be reduced or eliminated. The methods are simple, effective, and may be self-administered.

(2) Gravity. The most relentless and ultimately fatal stressing force in the human experience is the force of gravity. Using simple new methods and equipment, the debilitating effects of the force of gravity may be greatly reduced, and gravity itself used to help stem or reverse the aging process.

(3) Nutrition. Research has revealed certain simple but far-reaching changes in diet, coupled with exercise, can open the body to a vastly enhanced experience of its own remarkable therapeutic and recuperative powers, and its naturally extended longevity.

The Club's simple program, using simple equipment and methods, based on the simple principles outlined above, may be brought directly into the average home at a cost the average person can afford.

It is the purpose of the One Hundred Plus Club to accomplish this objective both in the United States and abroad. To accomplish this objective, an effective advertising campaign and sales force are needed.

Once that purpose is well along toward successful accomplishment, another goal of the Club is the establishment of Longevity Headquarters-- Total Health Headquarters-- in major cities to serve as organizational centers for the Club's varied activities. These activities will include travel and adventure programs, special instruction and training in many different areas of life enhancement, along with special health training and experiences and therapies, including psychological.

A third plan calls for the establishment, under the supervision of medical and

and other professional health groups, of Longevity Clinics that will be professionally administered.

Fourth, the Club intends to market Longevity Centers, to be established in corporate and other offices, as well as in health clubs, sports centers, etc. (These will contain the basic equipment, or more, but the Club will not be involved in supervision of the operation unless specifically requested to be.)

Each Metropolitan Headquarters will be responsible for marketing and operating Longevity Clinics and Centers in its area.

Finally, there will also be a separate mail-order membership operation to reach those who are not readily accessible in the other operations, and to enable them to participate at varying levels of effectiveness.

Basic Elements of Club Membership At-Home

(1) A Psychological Program Via Cassette Tapes. These cassettes will remove the unhealthy, negative, death-directed aspects of a member's psychological and subconscious programming. They employ a combination of medical hypnosis, mind-power methods, creative mental focusing, visualization, and affirmations. Two cassettes per month will be supplied during the first year, with special supplements as needed thereafter. They also create highly positive, life-affirming mental attitudes in users.

(2) One Rebounder. This device is, in effect, a mini-trampoline for use in the home. Consistent use of this device has an astonishingly beneficial effect on the human body. These effects are based on how the body's basic systems, down to the cellular level, react to and are strengthened by changing gravitational stress, and acceleration and deceleration stresses. The impact is especially profound on the vital lymphatic system as well as on the capillary system and heart. This device replaces, in a demonstrated superior fashion, virtually every other exercise modality, including jogging and jumping rope. It is capable of being used by almost anyone in almost any condition except bedridden. It is inexpensive (retail: under $200). And it is highly enjoyable to use. Unlike most exercises, people really enjoy rebounding and look forward to their next session. Studies indicate it is the most efficient, effective exercise yet devised. Commercially available.

(3) The Gravity Guiding System. This remarkable invention, created by the leading medical authority on back problems, who is also a pioneer and authority in the therapeutic uses of physical exercise, produces far-reaching and often miraculous results in a surprisingly short time through inversion-- reversing and varying the body's experience of the force of gravity. This device is easy to use and also enjoyable. Commercially available in two models. (The least expensive one, the portable model, retails at $795.)

September 24, 2013

The One Hundred Plus Club- 3

(4) <u>Nutritional Guidance System</u>. Adapted from its medical program, the Total Person Institute offers a computer analysis of individual dietary plus supplement needs, yielding precise nutritionally balanced programs for individual dietary requirements for maximum health and wellbeing. This program offers the optimum scientific approach to knowing precisely what your body needs for maximum health and longevity, eliminating all toxic and other dysfunctional inputs. Commercially available, but some adaptation to Club purposes required. (Costs: Home urine/saliva analysis kit, under $200, for family use. Regular computer analyses and recommendations: under $50 per person per year-- including eight separate individual analyses and guidance reports.)

(5) <u>Superlongevity Home Instruction Program.</u> The educational part of Club membership includes a monthly newsletter and manuals and carefully selected books on health, diet, exercise, psychology, prosperity and success. Among the manuals and books: Dr. Clark Cameron's *Superlongevity Instruction Manual,* Dr. Robert Martin's *The Gravity Guiding System*, Albert Carter's *The Miracles of Rebound Exercise*, Dr. Peter Cranford's *How To Be Your Own Psychologist,* plus several outstanding volumes on dieting for long and happy life. (Dr. Cameron's *How to Live to Be One Hundred Plus!*, now in preparation, will also be included when it is published.)   Also: Susan Smith Jones' *The Main Ingredients: Positive Thinking, Exercise & Diet,* and Adelaide Bry's *Visualization.*

      *   *   *   *   *   *

Present plans call for selling a ten-year program with a three-year payout on membership. $495 Initiation Fee plus $10 per week plus separate charges on the TPI Individual Nutrition Guidance Program, for more than one person. (Preliminary estimates.)

<u>Current Status</u>

All the elements of this program either exist in commercial form or can be brought into commercial form within several months at a modest investment.

The enterprise is now ready to be capitalized and for a business marketing organization to be brought into being to carry out the Phase One plan.

A pro forma marketing plan is being prepared on the Phase One Direct Sales program.

Next stages of development include:

(A) $300,000 loan for developmental capitalization.
(B) Going to the stockmarket for operating capital, from which the initial loan will be repaid.
(C) Beginning operations in maximum-opportunity test markets.

NOTE: Supplemental page follows.

NOTES:

(6) <u>Additional or Superior Equipment.</u>

The following will be among the add-ons available at time of signing up for Club membership, or later:

(a) <u>Additional Rebounder(s)</u>. The ideal combination is one for home, one for the office. Perfect instead of a Coffee Break. Ideal before lunch to tone down or replace appetite for food. Also great in case you miss your morning exercise session at home. And makes the greatest gift imaginable for parents (especially aging ones, or ones with the kinds of problems it helps) and friends-- or anyone!

(b) <u>Installation Model of Gravity Guiding System.</u> Much more complete range of exercises is possible with this original model. Provides the ideal home gymnastic set-up. Everything the portable model offers, plus much, much more. (Retail: $1195.)

(c) <u>Additional Gravity Inversion Boots</u>. Great for friends, relatives as an introduction to the inversion experience. (Retail: $80.)

(d) <u>Chinbars</u>. For use with boots. Special instructions on how to rig for hanging upside down and swinging stresses.

(e) <u>Total Gym</u>. The perfect all-purpose home body conditioning and development unit. Works completely with (and against) the force of gravity. Whatever can be done at a Nautilus or Health Spa gym, you can do simply and effectively and much more enjoyably, in your home with this extraordinary device. (Retail: $695.)

(d) <u>Dynavit</u>. The best available aerobic-control exercise device on the market. A computerized exercycle that provides ongoing readouts on your aerobic requirements and pulse levels, monitored in accordance with age, weight, and sex norms. Provides current age (physiological) measure based on your condition. (Retail: $2250.)

(e) <u>Float-to-Relax or Samadhi Tank</u>. In terms of construction, very different units designed, however, to accomplish the same objective: most total relaxation available on planet earth. Float totally free of the most basic stresses to which the human body and mind are constantly subject: gravitational, biochemical, thermal, visual, auditory, proprioceptive. Cut your required sleeping time in half. Also idea for mental (subconscious) re-programming, and complete relief of mental stress. (Retail: Samadhi, $2,000; Float-to-Relax, $3,000.)

(f) <u>Bullworker</u>-- separate models for men and women. Ideal quick exerciser for body strength and muscle tone. The best inexpensive substitute for the Total Gym. (Retail: $35.)

(g) <u>Family Trampoline</u>. A superb addition to, or replacement for, the Rebounder. Several models available, retail $1500- 2500.)

(7) <u>Other Products and Services.</u>

(a) The Club can carefully select and private-label top lines of vitamins and other health foods and health supplements.

(b) The Club should develop its own line of T-shirts, running suits and shorts, sweatshirts, socks, all-weather hiking jackets, etc.

(c) As membership grows, the Club can start offering a variety of worthwhile supplementary services including group travel, adventure, etc.

Chapter 13.
How Long Will You Live?

WEBSITES & SURVIVOR TYPES

HOW LONG WILL YOU live? It depends on lifestyle habits and family DNA; experts say between 20 and 30 percent is determined by your genes.

In mid-August 2013, I went to three websites to get a current calculation. Since getting deeply into completing this book I've become re-energized to extend my longevity target date to age 105.

Sixteen months ago I believed I was good for about 94 years. However, in early 2013, after a 15 year suspension, I returned to my hatha yoga exercises and recumbent bike cycling regimen. Next, I switched to an herbal tea with stevia sweetener in lieu of coffee in the AM. Then, I added more veggies, fresh fruits, and nuts.

The website http://gosset.wharton.upenn.edu/mortality/ calculates life expectancy based on a questionnaire. My result in April of 2012 was to expect a lifespan of 92 ½ years. Since then, I'm 12 pounds lighter and I've implemented a healthier diet. 96.8 years is Gosset's new estimate for my lifespan, a four year gain from the previous questionnaire submission. In my opinion, this website is biased toward shorter lifespans. Note: Some on-line calculators don't ask if the subject person has been diagnosed with cancer or some other life shortening condition.

On the website http://www.peterrussell.com/Odds/VirtualAge.php my life expectancy is 98.6 years, and my virtual age is 71.4 (about 11 years less than my actual age).

The third site, http://media.nmfn.com/tnetwork/lifespan/#0 the Northwestern Mutual Calculator, is from the prestigious life insurance carrier. I was congratulated for my estimated 104 year life expectancy. This result is the closest to my re-set goal of 105. Averaging all three estimates gives me about a 50/50 chance of becoming a centenarian. Of course, since this is a mean, half of those like me will live longer and half will live less than the age number calculated.

Largely in the last decade, many professional life insurance under-writers and Certified Financial Planners (CFP) have helped mon-eyed clients better plan their family income, retirement, and gifting with this new methodology. Questions, such as, "Will my wealth last as long as my life?" have become easier to answer.

Financial planning is becoming more realistic for needs such as long term care policy provisions, busi-ness agreements, and divorce settle-ments. Each person's financial needs are different, so simply looking at life expectancy averages from mor-tality tables is misleading, if not a professional error. Savvy insurance company underwriters are skilled at looking at medical findings as well as lifestyle – exercise, diet, alcohol, occupation, smoking, and hobbies to determine the composite scoring.

We now know we can grow our brains at any age. It's primarily ex-ercise, diet, and stress reduction combined with the five remaining healthy habits that offer the likeli-hood of many more productive years of life. This is the mission of the 100 Plus Club.

What about super centenarians (110 plus life spans)?

A California *West County Times*, July 11, 2013, article cited a Walnut Creek, California man, James Fos-ter McCoubrey, who passed in July as the oldest man (just short of 112 years) in the world. Up until June of 2013, a Japanese man held that title. Mr. McCoubrey was born in St. John's, Newfoundland, Canada. Later, he moved to Massachusetts until school ended for him in the 8th grade. For years he was in the heating oil business and sold insurance as well. At age 95, he learned how to navigate the Internet. He loved to tell stories and embraced change.

Mr. McCoubrey's age was verified by Robert Young, a consultant for the *Guinness Book of World Records.* Mr. Young said that 90% of super centenarians are women. Of the current 56 oldest persons in the world (verified), 54 are women.

Dr. Leila Denmark, a pediatrician in the Atlanta, Georgia, area, died in 2012 at age 114. Dr. Denmark practiced medicine until age 110, and retired only because she was losing her vision. Her daughter, Mary Denmark, said she was otherwise well.

In early 2012, Dr. Denmark was one of only 89 super centenarians in the world. She didn't set out to become famous; her goal was to help raise healthy babies. Note: My wife, Betty Ann, was a patient of Dr. Denmark's, as were her grandchildren. Dr. Denmark was the first female pediatrician in the state of Georgia. Daughter Mary, her only child, is now 81. The dean of the Medical College of Georgia said she was one of the, "Oldest alums, and a shining example." She set the example to live right and eat right. "When you love what you do, it's not work, it's play" said her grandson, Steve Hutcheson of Atlanta.

Another Georgia gal, Besse Cooper of Monroe, died at age 116 in December of 2012. *The Atlanta Journal Constitution* reported she was a true record-breaker under the headline "Guinness Pays Tribute to Monroe Woman's Inspiring Longevity." In 2009, Besse said her secrets included, "I mind my own business and don't eat junk food." She lived on her own until age 105 according to her son, Sidney Cooper. She was named the world's oldest living person and Guinness noted, "Her 116 years and 100 days places her among the ten oldest (verified) people in history."

After all your good planning and the decision to live as long as possible by implementing the eight healthy habits, what about the unexpected – emergency situations or accidents? Do you know which of the five survivor personality types applies to you? Do you know the top three of twelve strengths you possess to survive? Do you know the best seat to be in during an airline crash landing? Statistically, the best place to have a heart attack? Do you know how long you have to escape a fire in a hotel, home, or vehicle? If not, I suggest you read the fascinating book by Ben Sherwood, *The Survivors Club*, and learn your survival type and strengths. Note: We recently heard from an emergency medical technician during a presentation about this book. He said, "The worst place to have a heart attack is the ER waiting room (of a local prestigious hospital)."

Afterword

by Sally Walker

UNCLE CHARLIE WAS A "natural" when it came to doing things that are considered healthy today, many decades after his death in 1958. He was health conscious because of his stomach problems, before the emphasis on preventative medicine and wellness became popular in the mainstream media during Uncle Charlie's final years. In fact, Dr. Paul Dudley White, Uncle Charlie's physician, was among the first proponents of exercise as a factor in disease prevention.

One example is eating organic. For every American of Uncle Charlie's era (1850-1958), organic food was the only type available. Inorganic fertilizers and pesticides were not mass marketed until the 1940s, when Uncle Charlie was already in his ninth decade of life.

Body Mass Index is a ratio based on a person's height and weight and is a simple method to determine if one's body weight is desirable. Un-

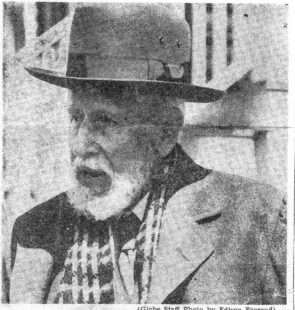

'Never Gave It a Thought; I Ran Like a Boy,' Says Youthful Centenarian

Belmont Man, 100, Sprints for Trolley

(Globe Staff Photo by Edison Farrand)
"NEVER FELT BETTER IN MY LIFE," says 100-year-old Charles W. Thiery of Belmont.

By EARL BANNER

Out in Belmont a few days back, Charles W. Thiery forgot himself. He chased—and caught —a trolley.

"I never gave it a thought at the time and I ran like a boy," Thiery said today. Mr. Thiery's running stint gains significance when one considers his age, 100 years and about 6 months.

He was born in Cambridge on Oct. 26, 1851, according to the records of the Cambridge City Clerk. He lived in Cambridge until eight or nine years ago, when he took up residence with two "youngsters," Mr. and Mrs.

L. Frank Merritt, 80 and 78, respectively, at 121 Hammond road, Belmont.

Thiery shows few signs of his age. His carriage is erect. His speech and movements are brisk. His handclasp is firm and strong. His eyesight is excellent, requiring the use of glasses only when he reads.

He still has 11 of his original teeth. The only wrinkles on his face are the marks of good humor at the corners of his eyes.

How does it feel to be '01? Mr. Thiery answers this with a very convincing: "I never felt better in my life."

THIERY Page 12

cle Charlie was a trim 115 pounds at 5'3", which is a body mass index rating of 20.4, a healthy weight. Go online to find a BMI calculator, get your number and then refer to the table below to see if you fall in the recommended range.

Body Mass Index (BMI) Ranges

Less than 18.50 = Underweight

18.50 to 24.99 = Healthy Weight

25.00 to 29.99 = Overweight

30 or more = Obese

Automats, the first fast food, started appearing in Uncle Charlie's region, the United States northeast, in the early part of the last century. However, fast food and franchised restaurants didn't start popping up in earnest until the 1950s, so Uncle Charlie was spared this temptation for most of his life. Keeping trim is a health as well as a quality of life issue.

The value of walking has been validated in study after study. Currently, walking, which was Uncle Charlie's daily habit, is considered a natural antidepressant. In the 1950s, Dr. White famously said, "A vigorous five-mile walk will do more good for an unhappy but otherwise healthy adult than all the medicine and psychology in the world." This practice kept him healthy and hardy, both physically and mentally, and can do the same for us.

"Stress Management" was not a wide-spread concept until the 1980s, so Uncle Charlie needed to rely on his own instinct to deal with life's challenges. In the business world, Uncle Charlie adapted himself to changes in the environment he had no control over, and as a result had several careers during his life. He was quoted a number of times saying, "Hard work don't kill a man." His interviews revealed a great sense of humor and someone who took things in stride. "I'm not one to fret," Uncle Charlie said. Through his work and efforts, he earned success, built his wealth, and was engaged with younger people because of his business connections. It's no wonder that Uncle Charlie didn't "feel old" until age 96!

Uncle Charlie kept his brain engaged by reading, following current events, and memberships in civic associations locally (Friendship Lodge of Odd Fellows, Cambridge), national (Massachusetts branch of the Republican Party), and worldwide (the Masons) to name a few. Uncle Charlie gave his time and treasure to his church, teaching Sunday school for decades and being their largest individual benefactor whose financial gift is still providing funding today.

"Boundaries" is a contemporary concept that Uncle Charlie applied in his day based on his Christian religious beliefs, which gave his life structure and purpose. Interviews indicate that Uncle Charlie did not "suffer fools gladly." He "shut the door" on people that he didn't respect and couldn't help.

Through these methods, Uncle Charlie kept his mind and body sharp. In summary, he was ahead of his time, not only in length of life, but quality of life as well. As the medium, Tom Flynn, noted, he's looking down on us with a twinkle, glad that because of this book, he's continuing to be a positive influence on family and others.

Bibliography

Alexander, Eben MD. *Proof of Heaven*. 2012. In a coma for seven days, Dr. Alexander, a neurosurgeon for 25 years, had a near death experience (NDE) that changed his beliefs about the spirit world. This book provides answers to skeptics, hope for those fearing death, and comfort to those who have lost loved ones.

Batchelder, Joshua H. CGA. *Personality Profiling in 90 Seconds*. 2006. The art of identifying a person's dominant character traits that aid understanding and acceptance of one's self and others.

Beaudine, Bob. *The Power of Who*. 2009. You already know everyone you need to know. You'll no longer obsess about networking and you'll pay more attention to those you know who'll support your destiny.

Buettner, Dan. *The Blue Zones*. 2008. Nine lessons for living longer from the people who've lived the longest.

Edward, John. *Afterlife*. 2003. Answers from the other side will guide you into gaining benefits from the spirit world. This book may help you find peace after losing loved ones and aid your search for your purpose while on earth.

Fuller, John Grant Jr. *The Airmen Who Would Not Die*. 1980. This book chronicles the true story of the English dirigible (airship) that crash landed in France in 1930. Eileen Garrett, a prominent Irish medium, connected many in the spirit world with their survivors. In addition, she relayed highly technical information. This tragedy was a case studied by Duke University researchers headed by psychologist J. B. Rhine, and also by the British Psychic Society. Evidence was recovered by medium Garrett using her methods without detectable fraud.

Franklin, Steve, Ph.D and Adler, Lynn Peters. *100: The Wisdom of American's Centenarians*. Wisdom and advice from those who have a lot of miles on their odometers.

Green, Jane Nugent, MS, BA. *You and Your Private I, Personality and the Written Self Image*. 1975. Graphological analyses focused on the personal pronoun I. Insights about a scripter's ego and issues with the subject's mother and father are identified. The PPI is also a special key to understanding a person's self-image.

Haldane, Bernard. *How to Make a Habit of Success*. 1975. Identify your talents by looking back to experiences you enjoyed during your youthful days. They're often overlooked but should be applied to help you achieve success and happiness.

Hittleman, Richard. *Be Young With Yoga.* 1972. This book details a 7-week course to stimulate your body to enjoy the vitality of youth. It was written by a famous TV yoga instructor.

Jacobs, Ruth Harriet. *Be An Outrageous Older Woman.* 1998. An action guide for women 50 and beyond from the prize-winning syndicated columnist and author.

Lindeman, Bard. *Be An Outrageous Older Man.* 1998. An action guide for men 50 and beyond.

Page, Eileen M. MGA. *The Paradox of Perfection.* 2001. Eileen explores all sides including the tyranny, curse, cost, quest, cult, and spirituality of perfection. This book can provide insight and comfort for those chasing perfectionism.

Pollan, Michael. *Food Rules: An Eater's Manual.* 2009. A practical approach to healthy shopping and eating without having to adhere to complicated plans and restrictions.

Sherwood, Ben. *The Survivors Club.* 2009. The producer of Good Morning America parades a rich collection of survivors' stories and insights. It relates fascinating tales of individuals surviving everything from airline crashes to jumping off the Golden Gate Bridge. It's a guide to help you determine your personality survivor type and the strengths that enable you to escape injury or death.

Simring, Sue Klaven & Steven S. *The Compatibility Quotient.* 1990. Who will stay married and who won't? Questionnaires and statistics help individuals and couples assess their relationships.

Sinetar, Marsha. *Do What You Love, the Money Will Follow.* 1989. Pursuing your talents leads to success and happiness.

Somers, Suzanne. *Bombshell.* 2012. Explosive medical secrets that will redefine aging are explained. Suzanne took the time and money to find the latest and best health strategies to live long and well.

Steadman, Alice. *Who's the Matter With Me?* 1981. The well-known author, artist and daughter of a 3rd generation physician compiles stories of miraculous medical recoveries from illnesses and accidents. Healing comes from identifying and correcting unresolved problems within interpersonal relationships. For example, when Uncle Charlie "came in from the outside" to help his father, his stomach problems began. While his father was his mentor, they often clashed. Would you think that if Uncle Charlie had this new knowledge he'd been able to end or relieve his digestive malady?

Stern, Sue Ellen. *He Just Doesn't Get It*. 1999. Simple solutions to the most common relationship problems are proposed. Author of *Loving An Imperfect Man*.

Stern, Jess. *Yoga, Youth and Reincarnation*. 1971. A suspicious, cynical New York City reporter travels to a Concord, Massachusetts ashram to uncover a sham. What he discovered are the many benefits of a hatha yoga regimen – new physical energy, mental focus, and spiritual growth.

Tan, Zaldy, MD, MPH. *Age-Proof Your Mind: Detect, Delay and Prevent Memory Loss – Before It's Too Late*. 2005. The book features a memory test and 60 minute brain workout.

Weil, Andrew MD. *Why Our Health Matters*. 2009. A vision of medicine that can transform our future. Understand American medicine, alternative lifestyles, and health care to achieve optimum health.

About the Authors

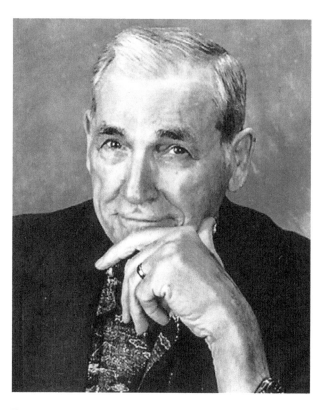

Josh Batchelder, CGA

Certified Graphoanalyst®, Analyst, Author, Lecturer, Teacher and Entertainer. Since 1976, providing business and private handwriting services: employment screening, comprehensive individual analyses, business and personal compatibility studies, and career cultivation counseling. Memberships: International Graphonanlysis Society (IGAS), South Eastern Handwriting Analysts (SEHA), American Handwriting Analysis Foundation (AHAF), American Assocation of Handwriting Analysts (AAHA). Pubications: *The Wheel: The Art of Wheel and Handwriting Analyses* (2011), *Quick & Insightful Personality Profiling* (2010), *Personality Profiling in 90 Seconds* (2006) and *Handwriting Reveals You* (2003). Since 1999, Josh has been a guest lecturer for the Celebrity, Princess, Royal Caribbean, and Norwegian cruise lines.

Insurance, Investments, and Financial Services. Chartered Life Underwriter (CLU), Chartered Financial Consultant (ChFC) and member, Atlanta Chapter of the National Society of Financial Service Professionals (since 1982). Multi-year Million Dollar Round Table (MDRT®) qualifier.

Military Service/Aviation. U.S. Air Force, Lt. Colonel, retired, 5000+

flying hours including 10 years (1962-1972) flying worldwide airlift missions, Chief Wing Navigator. Instrument Rated, Mission Qualifed Search & Rescue Pilot. Memberships: 59th Fighter Squadron Association (FSA), Air Force Navigator/Observer Association (AFNOA), Civil Air Patrol, PDK Senior Squdron, Atlanta Chapter of the Silver Wings Fraternity (SWF). Publications: *Climb to 8 and Wait* (2013), *Black Watch Diary – A Sequel* (2009), *Black Watch Diary* (2008).

Education and Civic Associations: Josh is a graduate of Harvard University with an AB in Social Relations (Social Psychology, Sociology, Small Group Dynamics). Certified Toastmaster, TM International. Tucker Business Association, and over 25 years with the Kiwanis.

Sally A. Walker

Livelihood. Like Charles Wesley Thiery, Sally has experience in a broad range of business and social activities. A graduate of Elmhurst College where she studied finance

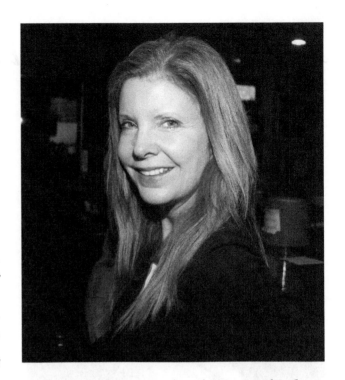

and economics, she has worked as a programmer/analyst in corporate America for over 10 years. Sally has served on numerous boards as a volunteer in her community.

Health and Wellness. During her college years, Sally supported herself by working as a certified aerobics instructor and personal trainer at health clubs in Chicago, Illinois. For five years (2002-2007) Sally taught weight loss and nutrition as she successfully coached clients to feel and look their best. Sally was a competitive tennis player for decades and is currently a social dancer.

.

CPSIA information can be obtained at www.ICGtesting.com
Printed in the USA
LVOW02s2257110614

389541LV00001B/1/P